the bone broth miracle diet

Erin Skinner, MS, RD, CPT

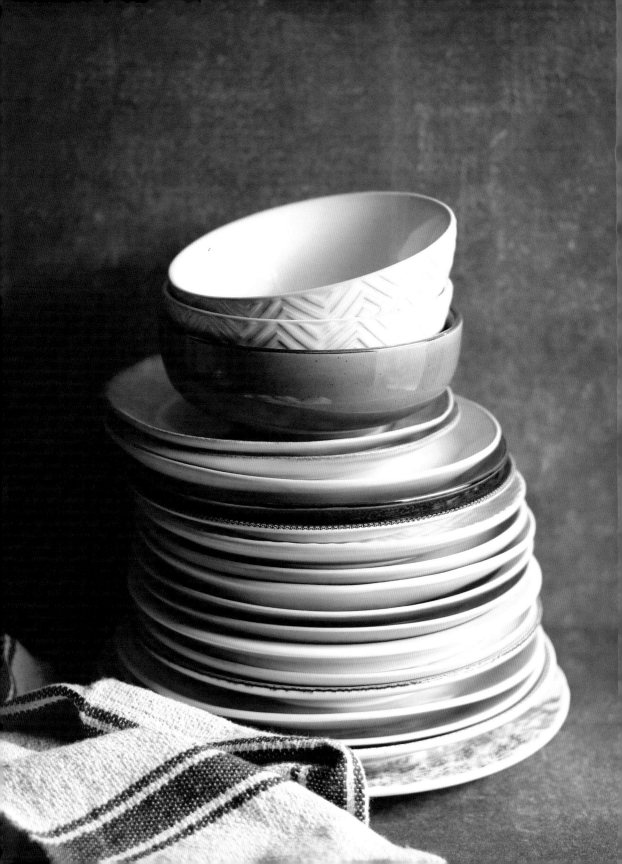

the bone broth miracle diet

Lose Weight, Feel Great, and Revitalize Your Health in Just 21 Days

Erin Skinner, MS, RD, CPT

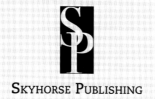

Skyhorse Publishing

All inquiries should be addressed to Skyhorse Publishing, 307 West 36th Street, 11th Floor, New York, NY 10018.

Skyhorse Publishing books may be purchased in bulk at special discounts for sales promotion, corporate gifts, fund-raising, or educational purposes. Special editions can also be created to specifications. For details, contact the Special Sales Department, Skyhorse Publishing, 307 West 36th Street, 11th Floor, New York, NY 10018 or info@skyhorsepublishing.com.

Skyhorse® and Skyhorse Publishing® are registered trademarks of Skyhorse Publishing, Inc.®, a Delaware corporation.

Visit our website at www.skyhorsepublishing.com.

10 9 8 7 6 5 4 3 2 1

Library of Congress Cataloging-in-Publication Data is available on file.

Cover design by Jane Sheppard
Cover photo by iStockphotos
Recipe photos and photos on pages 2 and 44 by Allan Penn
All other photos by iStockphotos

ISBN: 978-1-5107-1854-8
eBook ISBN: 978-1-5107-1855-5

Printed in China

table of contents

Acknowledgments

I am extremely grateful to my incredible husband Tom for his help and support in writing this book. Tom, you have made enormous sacrifices to support my career as a dietitian and to allow this book to become a reality. It would not have been possible without you, and I am very thankful.

I also send thanks to my incredible clients who inspire and teach me and who bravely piloted this program. I am wishing you all the best.

Thank you to my incredible family for supporting and teaching me. I find that some people can be scientific-minded clinicians and that some people can cook and create recipes. Not many can do both. I have been blessed with an incredible combination of parents who perfectly equipped me for this work. My father Ken is a brilliant engineer who always made me feel like I am capable of anything. My mother Priscilla is a gifted artist who taught me to cook with creativity. I cannot express how grateful I am to you both. I also owe a huge debt of gratitude to my Grandma Paizs who taught me the value of good cooking and hard work.

This book also would not have been possible without the endless love and support that I receive from my in-laws, Mike and Pam, and my sisters, Laurel and Kelley. Thank you for the encouragement and support that you have provided in many ways.

One of the most precious gifts that I have ever received is the ability to write. I thank Mr. Sanchez for that precious skill and for the confidence that you have in me.

To Monica of Hollan Publishing, thank you for your support and for being such a joy to work with.

Finally, I thank my two young boys, Evan and Austin. Although you make it hard to find time to write a book, you ultimately make it possible. You are the absolute inspiration and motivation for everything I do.

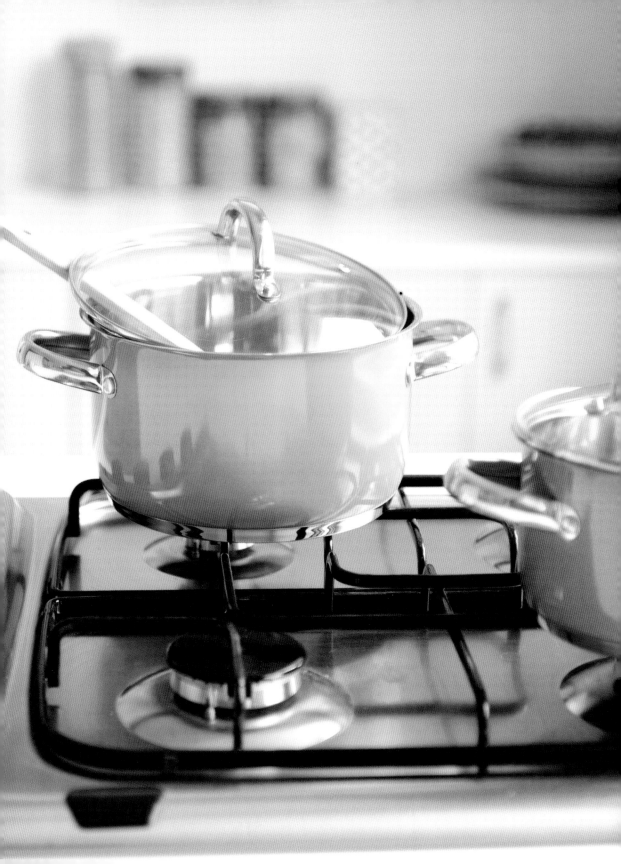

Introduction

Bone broth is everywhere lately. It's on restaurant menus, for sale online, found in health food stores, and is offered by the company that provides my organic produce box. I've even seen it for sale from food trucks in major cities. So, are there true benefits?

I find that there is a paucity of good information available regarding bone broth. Therefore, I've done a deep dive on the topic, so that I could provide you with the straight facts. It's true that bone broth is an incredible, healing food. When we combine it with a well-designed ancestral diet, we *really* have something powerful.

A bone broth-based ancestral diet is exactly what I've created in this book, and I can't wait for you to see what three weeks can do. If you are ready to commit to following this program for twenty-one days, then here are the benefits you can expect:

- Increase insulin sensitivity
- Decrease inflammation
- Lose body fat
- Improve gut health and digestion
- Strengthen your joints, hair, skin, and nails
- Improve your mood, sleep, and energy

However, I'd like to warn you about something. If you're new to the world of ancestral health, then you might be in for some surprises. This program goes against a lot of the nutrition advice that you've heard for years. Here are some myths about nutrition that you may have heard:

- Saturated fat and dietary cholesterol are bad for you
- You should eat a low-fat diet
- You should eat more processed polyunsaturated fats such as canola, vegetable, corn oil, or margarine
- You should eat several servings of whole grains each day
- Salt is bad for you
- Breakfast is the most important meal of the day

- You shouldn't eat meat
- You should never eat carbohydrates
- You should eat lots of carbohydrates—every meal and snack
- Everyone should be eating/drinking lots of dairy for bone health
- You need to fast all day to get the benefits of intermittent fasting
- You need to take dietary supplements to lose weight and/or get healthier

If you find this surprising, just think about how the common nutrition advice is working for us—we are experiencing epidemic rates of obesity, diabetes, cancer, autoimmune diseases, depression, anxiety, asthma, osteoporosis, and heart disease. Even children are experiencing rising rates of obesity, early puberty, ADHD, autism, and type II diabetes. All of these diseases and conditions are nutrition-related.

We've gone terribly wrong with regard to nutrition. Ancestral nutrition is simply a way of correcting back to eating the foods our body was designed to expect. We thrive on this approach. I've seen hundreds of my clients experience life-changing results. So, give bone broth and ancestral nutrition a chance. You'll see firsthand why this approach is so effective.

I'll be providing more information about bone broth, ancestral diets, and intermittent fasting as we go on. Then, I combine these powerful principles in a twenty-one day program: The Bone Broth Miracle Diet. If you want to get started with the program right away, feel free to skip ahead to Chapter 8, then go back and read the earlier chapters once you're rolling. If you'd like all the background information first, then read the chapters in order. Let's get started!

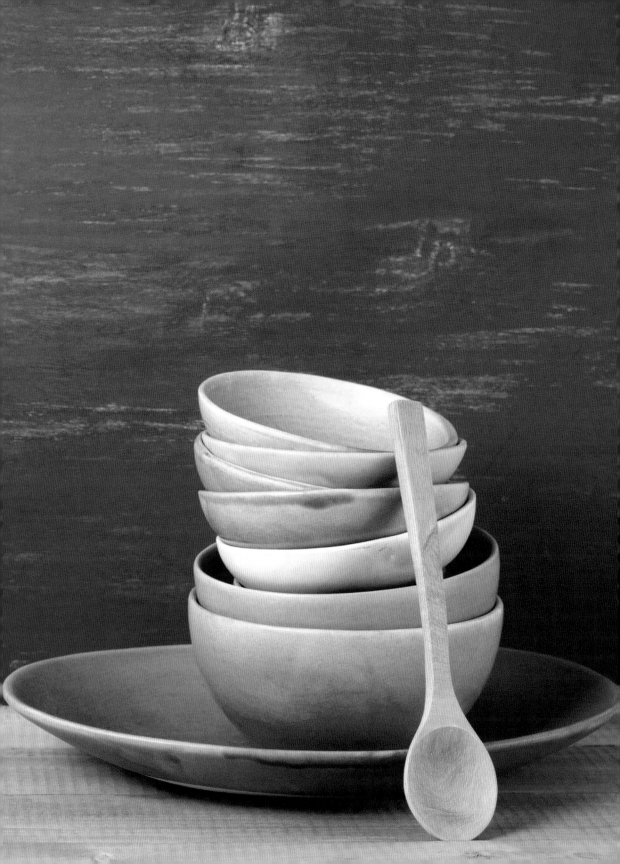

PART I

Why Bone Broth Is a Big Deal

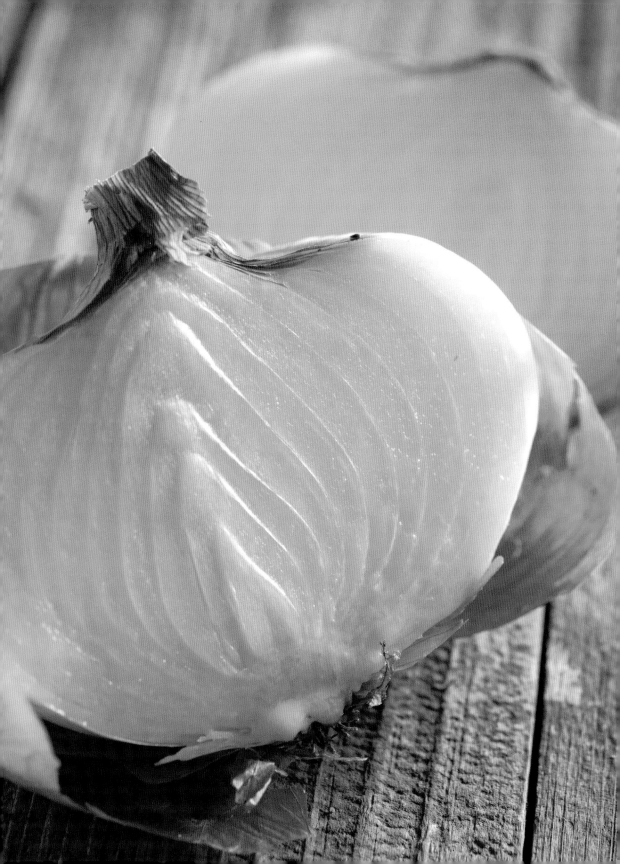

1

An Ancient Food

Because of your interest in bone broth, you are probably aware of the great irony of our time. Although we are becoming more advanced in many areas such as technology and transportation, our health is degrading. While we are much less likely than previous generations to die of infectious disease, we are now significantly *more* likely to experience chronic disease.

For example, two-thirds of Americans are overweight or obese. Even a quarter of children and adolescents are now overweight in the developed world. Along with this "obesity epidemic" comes a record-breaking incidence of related chronic diseases. These include cardiovascular disease, diabetes, hypertension, and cancer. Not coincidentally, these weight-related chronic diseases are the top causes of death in Western societies such as the United States.

At the same time, though many "modern humans" are overweight, they are also undernourished. Most consume foods that are high in calories yet low in nutrients. For example, a 2015 study published in *The American Journal of Clinical Nutrition* found that 76 percent of calories purchased by Americans are from processed foods and beverages. The vast majority of calories in these processed foods come from a small list of nutrient-poor ingredients: sugar, corn, soy, and refined flour. As a result, between 97 and 99 percent of American adults fall short of recommended nutrient intakes. Despite an overabundance of calories, modern diets commonly fall short of vitamins A, C, D, and E, calcium, magnesium, potassium, and vitamin K. These nutrients are essential for health and are vastly underconsumed in the modern world. We are starving in a sea of processed food.

The real problem here is that modern diets look nothing like those that humans consumed for the vast majority of our existence. Thus, there is a mismatch between what we eat and what our bodies are designed to expect. The problem is somewhat like putting diesel fuel in a car designed for unleaded. Just as that car wouldn't make it far down the road, modern humans are experiencing break downs in health. Despite medical advances, the life expectancy of some demographics of "Westerners" is decreasing for the first time since the government started keeping record. Western societies are actually experiencing *increasing* incidences of the following diet-related chronic diseases and conditions:

- Obesity
- Cardiovascular disease
- Cancer
- Autoimmune diseases (such as celiac, rheumatoid arthritis, type I diabetes, Hashimoto's thyroiditis, lupus, and inflammatory bowel disease)
- Type II diabetes
- Asthma
- Depression and anxiety
- ADHD
- Autism
- Osteoporosis

In fact, epidemiological studies estimate that the incidence of diabetes will double by 2015, and that the incidence of ADHD, Alzheimer's, diabetes, and cancer will *triple* by then. Autoimmune disease now effects 8 percent of modern populations, and is increasing by 12 to 15 percent annually. Judging by this rise of diet-related medical conditions, our diets are clearly not on point. The question is: *What* actually constitutes a healthful or "correct" diet?

The field of nutritional science is still fairly young, and there is an incredible amount of debate and conflicting evidence surrounding this topic. I have found that the most helpful way to consider what fits in a diet is to use an ancestral lens. In other words, consider if the food was a part of ancestral diets or if it is a new food.

This ancestral lens helps weed through the confusion surrounding food. Our species lived on ancestral foods for around 200,000 years. Then, around 10,000 years ago, everything changed with the agricultural revolution. The period since then has been a relative blink of the eye in human history. So, when we try to wade through what is right-versus-wrong to eat, it is essential to consider whether that food was historically a part of our diets or if it is a new introduction.

The importance of this ancestral perspective cannot be over-emphasized. Some of the Neolithic foods in our diet include wheat, soy, corn, and refined sugar. These foods constitute the *majority* of the calories consumed in modern societies.

Thus, our current diet is completely unlike anything our species has encountered before. No wonder we are experiencing a meltdown of modern health!

Bone broth actually serves as an example of how our diets have transitioned away from the ancestral template. Although bone broth is popular at the moment, it was recently a nearly forgotten food.

Bone broth (or stock) is actually an ancient food. It was an effective, efficient staple of our hunter-gatherer ancestors for centuries. It is an efficient use of food when supplies are scarce. It provides incredible health benefits. Not to mention, it contains delicious free glutamates.

Free glutamates provide the savory "umami" flavor we all love. Have you ever wondered why restaurant food tends to taste better than home-cooked food? This is in large part thanks to free glutamates being readily available in commercially made food. This adds an umami flavor and enhances the taste.

Unfortunately, something went horribly wrong with free glutamates back in 1959 when the FDA classified the food additive monosodium glutamate (MSG) as "generally recognized as safe" (GRAS). Up until that point, broth was widely used to flavor and nourish foods. However, with the introduction of monosodium glutamate (MSG), broth went out of favor.

The safety of MSG can be argued either way. Although it is a neurotoxin for mice, there is no conclusive evidence that it is harmful for humans. That being said, some people do experience a phenomenon colloquially known as "Chinese Restaurant Syndrome" when they consume it. The symptoms include headaches, flushing, sweating, numbness, chest pain, nausea, heart palpitations, and weakness. Interestingly, these symptoms are not experienced when natural glutamates are consumed—they only occur with MSG.

Aside from the possible risks of MSG consumption, the additional problem is that the low cost and instant availability of MSG marginalized bone broth in the modern diet. MSG is found under a variety of names and is added to commercially available soups, condiments, sauces, bouillon, and stock. Even the stock used in restaurants usually begins with a commercial soup base made with MSG rather than real bones.

While MSG is well-tolerated by many, the real tragedy here is that its widespread use caused broth to become an old-fashioned memory. The incredibly important, healing components of real bone broth were lost. It seems that we haven't benefited by switching from real broth to artificial food additives. As a case in point, chicken bone broth has been shown to have anti-inflammatory and immune-supporting properties that are not present in commercially produced chicken soups. In fact, many of the conditions that real bone broth helps prevent and heal are now seen in the highest prevalence in recorded medical history.

The change from broth to MSG was just one of many substitutions away from traditional diets that have occurred since the agricultural revolution. In fact, modern meals barely resemble those that we consumed for the vast majority of our existence. Western nations are paying the price with increasing incidence of diet-related chronic diseases.

Clearly we have gone horribly wrong somewhere.

The truth is that there is ancient wisdom in traditional diets. For eons, humans co-evolved with the existing food supply. As a result, our genes and physiology aligned to function optimally with consumption of those foods. Departure from this well-established model almost immediately resulted in epidemics of chronic disease in the Western world.

In fact, we can see this phenomenon in real time. As Western-style diets become more popular across the globe, each new nation that adopts them predictably begins to experience increased rates of these modern diseases. Only by going back to traditional diets can we regain our wellness. The reintroduction of bone broth is an important part of that transition.

2

Beneficial Components

Broth is a very complex, fascinating substance. Unfortunately, it has not been well researched. Frustratingly, this is the norm for foods that can't be patented like medications; the research dollars just aren't there. Additionally, creating identical batches of broth that satisfy scientific rigor is nearly impossible, and this further complicates the issue.

However, there is good evidence for the benefits of the compounds *within* bone broth. These compounds are the amino acids, fats, minerals, and proteoglycans that come from the cartilage, bone marrow, and mineralized bone in the broth.

Amino Acids

The protein building blocks, amino acids, found in broth are the most important component. When we consume proteins from animal cartilage and bone, we literally gain the building blocks required to support, heal, and grow our own bodies.

However, we have been led to believe a half-truth that makes this concept somewhat confusing. The half-truth is that, of the twenty amino acids, only nine of them are essential—that we can simply make the other eleven. In fact, we cannot easily generate the "non-essential" amino acids, especially in the presence of certain factors:

- High demand (i.e. athletes, growth, pregnancy, lactation, injury/burns)
- Low protein intake or poor protein digestion/absorption
- Lack of quality (animal) protein
- Sickness and disease
- Common nutrient deficiencies
- Advanced age
- Certain genetic polymorphisms (some gene mutations of our DNA do not allow us to perform the conversion between amino acids well)

In fact, many biochemists and clinical researchers believe that some of the eleven "nonessential" amino acids should be considered "conditionally essential." This means that in many situations people actually *do* need to obtain these amino acids in their diet. Some of these situations include acute or chronic illness, injury, poor adrenal function, nutrient deficiencies, and poor gastrointestinal/digestive function. Interestingly, the three most abundant amino acids in bone broth (glycine, proline, and glutamine) are among these "conditionally essential" amino acids.

The synthesis of proline, for example, only occurs in intestinal tissue, which means it requires a healthy intestinal metabolism. Unfortunately, poor gut health is extremely common. Thus, bone broth provides proline in the frequent case where it is essential due to inadequate production in the gut.

Even without poor intestinal metabolism, conditional amino acids cannot be generated from other amino acids very well. Studies have found that when healthy males consume a diet devoid of proline, their plasma levels of proline drop by 22 percent.

In another example, diets lacking the amino acids proline and glutamic acid significantly slow growth in baby rats. It seems that these "nonessential" amino acids are essential in some cases, and that they cannot be simply created when they are absent from the diet. Both of these amino acids, proline and glutamine, are among the most abundant in bone broth.

So, bone broth provides amino acids that are essential to obtain from dietary sources. Not only are these amino acids "conditionally essential," they are *not* widely available from dietary sources other than bone broth. As I will explain in further detail, the best sources of these amino acids are the animal parts that are not usually eaten in the modern world. Thus, bone broth provides the "missing link," so to speak.

As shown in Table 1, the four most abundant amino acids in bone broth are: glycine, proline, glutamine (glutamic acid), and alanine. Each has their own important story with regard to its benefits.

Glycine

The most abundant amino acid in bone broth is glycine, with around 1.7 grams per 8 oz serving. Aside from bone broth, the best dietary sources are gelatin, cured meats, and animal products such as pork skins, ears, and knuckles. Thus, glycine is primarily obtained from animal sources. Note that significant sources of glycine are *not* the parts of the animal usually consumed (muscle meat) but are the parts used in bone broth (skin, cartilage, and bone).

Amino Acids in Chicken Bone Broth (8 fl oz)

Amino Acids	Bone Broth (long-cooked) (mg)	Meat Stock (short cooked) (mg)
Glycine	1773.33	450
Glutamic Acid	1013.33	366.67
Proline	986.67	242.33
Alanine	773.33	214.33
Arginine	696.67	170.67
Aspartic Acid	553.33	161
Lysine	303	127.67
Histidine	93.67	98.67
Leucine	276.33	92.33
Serine	242.67	85.67
Threonine	214	70.33
Valine	181	63.67
Phenylalanine	192.33	56.67
Isoleucine	131.67	43
Tyrosine	76.33	34
Methionine	96.33	26.13
Cystine	24.03	23.77

The sample broth was prepared using organic chickens by Kim Schuette of Biodynamic Wellness and GAPSinfo.com. Analysis was performed by Covance Laboratories, Madison, Wisconsin.

Although gelatin is another high source of glycine, it is a riskier choice than bone broth. Great care must be taken with its sourcing. Gelatin is especially susceptible to contamination with glyphosate (the herbicide known as Roundup). This is because the molecular structure of glyphosate closely mimics glycine. The molecules are so similar that glyphosate actually replaces glycine in the proteins of organisms that are exposed to it. Because gelatin is high in glycine, it can contain elevated levels of glyphosate. In fact, gelatin is used in research as the vehicle for delivery of glyphosate to test subjects. Thus, although gelatin is a high source of glycine, it also comes with risk and must be carefully sourced.

Cured meats are another good source of glycine but, again, there are concerns. Cured meats have been associated with elevated risks of cardiovascular disease, diabetes mellitus, and some types of cancer.

Because of these concerns regarding commercially available gelatin and cured meats, bone broth using organic ingredients provides the cleanest source of readily absorbable dietary glycine.

As described previously, glycine is a conditionally essential amino acid. In fact, it is nearly impossible to endogenously produce the amount of glycine needed. The average production and dietary intake of glycine puts us around 10 grams short each day of what we require. This shortfall of glycine intake impacts the many important functions of glycine:

- Glycine is essential for synthesis of collagen for stronger bones, skin, joint cartilage, hair, and nails.
- It plays an important role in metabolism by stimulating the release of human growth hormone. This increases metabolic rate and stimulates the release of triglycerides from fat cells.
- It supports the detoxification functions of the liver.
- Glycine increases antioxidant reactions, which means that it decreases oxidative stress and helps fight cancer.
- It supports neurological function; glycine is an inhibitory neurotransmitter that inhibits norepinephrine, reducing anxiety and increasing calmness.
- Glycine increases energy by improving sleep quality and decreasing daytime fatigue.
- It supports wound healing.
- Glycine improves insulin sensitivity, which is essential for avoiding type II diabetes and metabolic syndrome.
- It supports maintenance of immune function, helping to avoid illness and the immune dysregulation found in autoimmune disease.
- Glycine is essential for the production of bile and, thus, dietary fatty acid digestion. This is significant considering the fact that most people are deficient in the fat-soluble vitamins A and D. Without proper fat absorption, these nutrients cannot be absorbed.

Thus, glycine is used to treat cancer, diabetes, obesity, cardiovascular disease, wounds, and osteoarthritis. Because our own body's production of glycine is insufficient, it is critical that we consume it from dietary sources.

Another extremely important point with regard to glycine is that it counteracts the damaging effects of excess methionine. Methionine is another amino acid, and there is a great body of evidence that it is especially susceptible to oxidation by reactive oxygen species (ROS). Oxidation is the underlying cause of aging and is associated with many common diseases: Alzheimer's disease, respiratory distress syndrome, muscular dystrophy, cataracts, rheumatoid arthritis, atherosclerosis, diabetes, Parkinson's disease, hypertension, cystic fibrosis, and ulcerative colitis. The effect of methionine and oxidation are so powerful that dietary restriction of methionine significantly extends lifespan. The oxidation of methionine is believed to be a significant reason why caloric restriction extends lifespan.

The average Western human does not limit methionine. In fact, intake is usually very high because muscle meat (such as chicken breast and steak) is a high source of methionine. Consuming large amounts of muscle meat and not getting enough glycine, renders an imbalance that contributes to harmful oxidative stress. Fortunately, glycine has been shown to alleviate methionine toxicity. This is because glycine is essential for clearance of excess methionine via the liver. Studies have shown that the addition of glycine to the diet rids the body of excess methionine, helping to restore balance.

It is important to note as well that methionine does serve important functions in the body. It is a precursor of glutathione, the master antioxidant of the body. It also supports cellular signaling, supports the liver's detoxification pathways, and aids in cellular growth and repair. So, methionine is important—when balanced properly. Thus, we see the intelligence of ancestral diets at work. The methionine supplied by muscle meats should be consumed in balance with the glycine provided by the skin and cartilage of the animal. By moving away from the "nose-to-tail" style of eating we once routinely practiced, we have created an imbalance of amino acids that increases our risk of oxidation and disease.

Glutamine

The second most abundant amino acid in bone broth is glutamic acid. Each 8-ounce serving contains around 1 gram of glutamic acid, which the body easily converts to glutamine. This is a fairly high source, considering that normal dietary intake of glutamine is 5–10 grams per day.

Glutamine is the most abundant amino acid in the body and is conditionally essential. It serves many important functions, including the maintenance of nitrogen balance, acid-base homeostasis, and regulation of glucose metabolism. During times of critical illness or injury, the body does not produce enough glutamine to meet needs. Athletes with a high training load also do not produce enough glutamine, and a deficiency of glutamine is a significant cause of overtraining syndrome. There is strong evidence that it helps in the cases of burns, critical illness, HIV/AIDS-related muscle wasting, chemotherapy-induced oral mucositis, and surgery.

It is critical to understand that when the body is stressed, glutamine needs exceed normal dietary intake. When the stress hormone cortisol is elevated, glucagon rises to stimulate gluconeogenesis, the production of glucose from non-carbohydrate sources. Gluconeogenesis requires glutamine to the degree that it literally becomes depleted by prolonged stress. This occurs when the body is stressed by disease, exercise, or injury.

Glutamine also serves as fuel for many important cell types: enterocytes (intestinal cells), renal (kidney) cells, neurons, immune cells, and pancreatic beta (insulin-producing) cells. Thus, any time that increased cell turnover is required, glutamine needs are increased. In fact, lack of dietary glutamine has been shown to result in apoptosis (cell death) of rapidly dividing cells. Although some theorize that this fact makes glutamine restriction a possible cancer treatment, the opposite is actually true. Glutamine has been shown to stimulate the activation of tumor suppression gene p53. These p53 proteins actually induce cancer cell death and tumor regression.

One area of the body that experiences the highest cell turnover is the mucosal lining of the gastrointestinal tract. The integrity of the tight junctions between the epithelial (gut lining) cells of the mucosa is extremely important. Lack of gut barrier function plays a major role in the symptoms caused by Irritable Bowel Disease (IBD), Irritable Bowel Syndrome (IBS), infectious enterocolitis, and celiac disease. Glutamine has been shown to repair and maintain gut barrier function. On the other hand, lack of dietary glutamine greatly hinders the growth of the intestinal epithelial cells.

There has been some controversy regarding whether glutamine should be used in the case of small intestinal bacterial overgrowth (SIBO), a common cause of IBS.

The theory here is that the glutamine will feed the bacteria in the small intestine, making the SIBO worse. There is no evidence to substantiate this theory though, and many people have experienced improvement of SIBO using glutamine. SIBO is associated with increased gut permeability, so glutamine should not be removed from consideration when it comes to SIBO treatment. IBS and/or SIBO should be treated under the guidance of a trained medical professional who can make a clinical decision regarding the use of glutamine and other treatment options.

Another critical function of glutamine is the maintenance of healthy immune function. Glutamine feeds lymphocyte immune cells and stimulates their proliferation. It also supports the production of the cytokines (messaging proteins) that stimulate immune cells to act. In fact, glutamine availability directly influences the action of macrophage immune cells. Because of its critical role in supporting the immune system, glutamine has been used to support the treatment of cancer, bone marrow transplants, and autoimmunity.

Glutamine (along with glycine and cysteine) also serves as an important substrate for glutathione, the master antioxidant. Glutathione acts as protection against oxidative damage by neutralizing free radicals. Thus, it plays an important role in reducing inflammation. It serves in the prevention and treatment of heart disease, alcoholism, cancer, HIV/AIDS, hepatitis, type II diabetes, Parkinson's Disease, and Alzheimer's Disease. Glutathione production decreases with age, when the risk of many of these diseases is highest and when protein intake usually decreases. Thus, glutamine intake is important to maintain or even increase with age.

There have been claims that glutamine can help reduce sugar cravings and thus aid weight loss. Studies have found that supplemental glutamine acts much like glucose to aid recovery from hypoglycemia (low blood sugar), although the opposite was true for type I diabetics. Some evidence shows that glutamine may improve insulin sensitivity. In fact, one pilot study did find that supplemental glutamine taken for 4 weeks resulted in significant weight loss and decreased waist size for non-dieting obese women. However, these women took ½ gram of glutamine per kilogram of body weight per day, which is significantly higher than the amount that bone broth contains.

Finally, glutamine plays an important role in the neurological system. It is the most abundant amino acid in the cerebrospinal fluid and a precursor for the inhibitory neurotransmitter GABA. It is also a precursor for the excitatory amino acid glutamate. Glutamine seems to also regulate production of the important messenger nitric oxide. Disturbances of glutamine availability, transport, or metabolism have been shown to play a role in epilepsy and hepatic encephalopathy. Glutamine has also been suggested as a "brain food" that can help improve depression, anxiety, and ADHD.

However, there is a double-edged sword when it comes to glutamine and neurology. Some studies find that when excess glutamate is produced, acute and chronic neurological diseases can result. Unfortunately, children with ADHD are more likely to be sensitive to glutamine. This glutamine intolerance is likely the mechanism behind the severe adverse reaction some people experience when they consume monosodium glutamate (MSG)—the reaction known as "Chinese Restaurant Syndrome." Thus it is wise to consume glutamine with caution. There is no evidence that the relatively small dose from bone broth will cause harm. In fact, glutamine is safe at extremely high doses in patients who are not sensitive. However, processed foods containing MSG should be avoided. Also, any large doses of supplemental glutamine should be taken under the guidance of a health professional.

Thus, glutamine is essential for a wide variety of important physiological functions: healthy cell proliferation, gut integrity, immune function, reducing inflammation, neurological functioning, and glucose metabolism. Oral intake should be increased when dietary protein intake is low or if the body is stressed, either physiologically or by tissue damage. Although some people are sensitive to glutamine, most people can consume it in high quantities. Bone broth provides this conditionally essential amino acid from a whole food source.

Proline

As for the amino acid proline, the greatest dietary sources are gelatin, pork skins, cheese, and soy protein isolates. Again, the safest choice is bone broth with 986.67 mg (nearly 1 gram) per 8-ounce serving. As described previously, proline is conditionally essential. Proline serum levels of test subjects who ate a proline-free diet dropped significantly. The generation of proline requires glutamine which, as described above, is often deficient. In addition to glutamine, vitamin C is required for proline to be converted to its active form, hydroxyproline. Unfortunately, vitamin C is underconsumed by many individuals.

Proline serves many important functions. Along with glycine, it is a critical building block for collagen, the body's major structural protein. Deficiencies of collagen result in bruising and in weakened ligaments, tendons, and blood vessels. Collagen is the protein that maintains integrity of the skin, and decreased collagen is associated with wrinkles and cellulite. Proline is also required for cartilage production and is therefore essential for joint health. It also supports wound healing, anti-oxidative functions (reducing inflammation), and supports the immune system. Proline has been found to be in high demand immediately following traumatic brain injury (TBI), and a compound containing proline has been shown to decrease the damage caused by TBIs.

As is the case with glycine and glutamine, modern diets are low in the animal parts that traditionally provided proline. Dairy and soy foods are modern sources of proline, but both come with concerns of their own. In the end, bone broth is the best choice for providing proline to support immunity, wound healing, lowered inflammation, and increased production of collagen and cartilage. I will go into more detail about the importance of collagen and cartilage as we go on.

Alanine

Alanine is the next most abundant amino acid in bone broth, at around 0.7 gram per 8-ounce serving. Alanine serves important functions in athletic performance (it is converted to pyruvate then lactate), maintenance of blood glucose, and immune function. Conversion to L-alanine, the form used in muscle tissue, requires the conditionally essential amino acid glutamine. However, alanine itself is available in abundance from other ancestral foods such as eggs and fish, so bone broth does not provide the only healthy source. Because it can be acquired from multiple sources, alanine is rarely deficient, with the exception being vitamin B_6 deficiency.

Nutrients

Although some falsely claim otherwise, bone broth is relatively low in vitamins and minerals. The most common nutrient claim that I see for bone broth is that it is high in calcium. Although the calcium content of bone broth does increase when it is cooked in acid (i.e. vinegar), the truth is that it still remains at a fairly low level. Thus, the healing properties of bone broth are more related to a synergy between the nutrients it does contain: minerals, amino acids, fats, and proteoglycans. Table 2 lists the mineral levels found in organic chicken bone broth. Similar values were found in older published studies.

Minerals in Chicken Bone Broth (8 fl oz)

Minerals	
Calcium	6.14 mg
Copper	<0.0298 mg
Iron	<0.119 mg
Magnesium	5.20 mg
Manganese	0.024 mg
Phosphorus	19.5 mg
Potassium	94.3 mg
Sodium	57.5 mg
Zinc	0.0517 mg

* The sample broth was prepared using organic chickens by Kim Schuette of Biodynamic Wellness and GAPSinfo.com. Analysis was performed by Covance Laboratories, Madison, Wisconsin.

Obviously, the mineral content of the broth will vary based on the type of bones that are used. Fish bones and egg shells degrade more fully when cooked in broth and will therefore likely release more minerals. The length of cooking time and the addition of acid to the cooking liquid are also important factors. For this reason, I include apple cider vinegar in the broth recipes of this program.

Sweet Molecules:
Glycoproteins and Amino Sugars

Here is where the benefits of bone broth literally start to come together. Bone broth contains several important types of glycosylated proteins known as proteoglycans. These are proteins attached to chains called glycosaminoglycans (GAGs), which contain many sugar molecules. Significantly, proteoglycans also contain a sulfate group. These important proteoglycans are used in connective tissue, joints, the gut lining, and even the immune system. They are not commonly found in foods but are abundant in bone broth as the broken-down components of the collagen and cartilage attached to bones. The most important of these "sweet molecules" in bone broth are glucosamine, chondroitin, hyaluronic acid, and N-acetylgalactosamine.

Glucosamine

One important component of the GAG chains of proteoglycans is glucosamine. It is used to build ligaments, cartilage, tendons, and the synovial fluid that cushions joints. Glucosamine is a glycoprotein (sugar + protein); it is composed of glucose and the amino acid glutamine. As previously stated, glutamine is conditionally essential; often our combined production and dietary consumption is less than our needs.

A further problem is that glucosamine requires a sulfur molecule (i.e., glucosamine sulfate). Unfortunately, sulfur is also lacking in our diets. One primary source of sulfur in the diet is sulfur-containing vegetables, which are largely underconsumed in modern diets. Examples of these vegetables include broccoli, cauliflower, Brussels sprouts, garlic, and onions. The second important source of sulfur is animal protein, which many people limit or avoid completely. Thus, lack of glutamine and sulfur causes glucosamine production to suffer. To make up for this, it is beneficial to take supplemental glucosamine.

Some of the specific benefits of glucosamine include:

- It has been shown by meta-analysis to significantly improve osteoarthritis symptoms compared to controls. It even improves symptoms more significantly than 3 grams per day of acetaminophen.
- It increases intestinal mucin secretion in a dose-dependent fashion. Inability to maintain this protective mucosal barrier (GAG layer) of the gut contributes to Inflammatory Bowel Disease (Crohn's Disease and Ulcerative Colitis), Peptic Ulcer Disease, and Interstitial Cystitis.
- It significantly decreases inflammation and symptoms of the autoimmune disease rheumatoid arthritis.

Chondroitin

Another important compound found in bone broth is a proteoglycan called chondroitin. Chondroitin is often sold in combination with glucosamine as a supplement for joint health. It is an essential component of cartilage. Just like with glucosamine, it requires the often-lacking sulfate group for it to function (i.e., chondroitin sulfate). Chondroitin sulfate offers the following benefits:

- The National Institutes of Health-sponsored GAIT (Glucosamine/Chondroitin Arthritis Intervention Trial) is a multi-center, double-blind, placebo-controlled clinical trial that compared glucosamine and chondroitin sulfate supplementation to the prescription medication Celebrex for treatment of knee osteoarthritis. The trial found that supplementation with glucosamine sulfate and chondroitin sulfate significantly reduced severe osteoarthritis pain as compared to controls. Glucosamine and chondroitin were even as effective as Celebrex for reducing symptoms in moderate to severe cases. These findings are especially significant considering that the FDA cites a two- to three-fold increased risk of heart attack or stroke with use of Celebrex.

- A 2012 comprehensive meta-analysis of placebo-controlled trials also found that chondroitin sulfate significantly reduces knee osteoarthritis symptoms.
- Injections containing chondroitin sulfate protect the eye during and after cataract surgery.
- Supplementation with chondroitin sulfate and hyaluronic acid reduces the rate of urinary tract infections (UTIs) among women with recurrent UTIs.
- Supplementation with glucosamine and chondroitin reduces C-reactive protein (CRP), a marker of inflammation, by 23 percent. This provides an explanation for the associated lower risk of colorectal and lung cancer with long-term use.

There is also some evidence that chondroitin can reduce the symptoms of dry eyes, exercise-induced muscle soreness, Gastroesophageal Reflux Disease (GERD), Interstitial Cystitis, Kashin-Beck Disease (a joint-destructive disease), psoriasis, urinary incontinence, and overactive bladder. It also may reduce the risk of myocardial infarction (MI) among those with a history of MI. However, more evidence is needed to conclusively show that chondroitin provides these benefits.

Hyaluronic Acid

Hyaluronic acid (HA) is a third important molecule in bone broth. It is a GAG composed of disaccharides (sugars). It forms huge proteoglycans that are found in connective, epithelial, and neural tissue. HA is unique among GAGs because it contains no sulfur molecule. The major function of HA is to hold water. It acts like a huge sponge molecule that holds water molecules where they are needed, such as between joints and in the skin. HA has an incredibly high turnover in the body, lasting only approximately three days. Bone broth provides HA in the forms of dissolved hyaline cartilage which comes from the ends of bones. So, unless we actually chew on the ends of bones, we do not get much HA in our diet. Although we can generate HA ourselves, there is evidence that supplementation helps in the following cases:

- It has been shown to improve skin moisture and even to stimulate the production of fibroblasts, the cells that create new connective tissue—fighting wrinkles from the inside out.
- Oral supplementation of HA reduces pain and increases function in osteoarthritis patients.
- It is an FDA-approved treatment for oral mucositis (stomatitis).
- HA improves the outcome of eye surgery for cataracts, corneal transplantation, lens implantation, and glaucoma.
- HA injections are an FDA-approved treatment for reducing facial wrinkles and folds.
- It is an approved intra-articular injection for treatment of osteoarthritis.
- HA aids healing of wounds, burns, and skin ulcers.

N-Acetylgalactosamine

Finally, N-acetylgalactosamine is an amino sugar found in bone broth. It is derived from the sugar molecule galactose, with an amino group attached. It is actually a component of the GAGs of chondroitin sulfate. Thus, it comes from the cartilage used in bone broth.

N-acetylgalactosamine serves as a component of many important glycolipid molecules, which means that it attaches to lipids. These glycolipids are incorporated into cell membranes and serve important messaging functions. Studies have found evidence that N-acetylgalactosamine plays a role in many important functions:

- Patients with coronary heart disease have lower amounts of N-acetylgalactosamine in their LDL cholesterol molecules, and this is associated with an increased accumulation of cholesterol in the cells of their arteries.

- It also is associated with improvement of joint damage and pain, to include injury, osteoarthritis, and rheumatoid arthritis. The molecule has been found to decrease the release of inflammatory oxidant molecules.
- N-acetylgalactosamine improves the blood flow and protective lining of the gastrointestinal tract and was shown to improve Crohn's Disease in children.
- It helps to protect against infectious disease such as the flu by supporting the messaging of the immune system.
- Alterations of N-acetylgalactosamine messaging have been connected to breast cancer.
- Finally, N-acetylgalactosamine was shown to decrease neurological autoimmunity. It is now being studied as a therapeutic approach to the autoimmune disease multiple sclerosis.

So, bone broth is pretty "sweet." It contains important sugar-containing molecules which are difficult to otherwise get in our diets. Some of these molecules include glucosamine sulfate, chondroitin sulfate, N-acetylgalactosamine, and hyaluronic acid (HA). The proteoglycans, GAGs, glycoproteins, and glycolipids produced using these molecules are important substrates for tissue repair, anti-inflammatory reactions, and immune function.

Collagen

If you've ever heard someone say that they are "falling apart" as they age, they aren't just exaggerating! Collagen, the "glue" that holds our body together, actually decreases and weakens with age. This loss of collagen is a pretty big deal when we consider that it provides structural function in all areas of the body:

- It maintains the integrity of the cartilage tissue that protects and cushions the joints.
- It holds bones and muscles together by strengthening ligaments.
- It maintains the integrity of the skin, preventing wrinkles, lines, and cellulite.
- It provides strength to hair and nails.
- It protects and maintains the gastrointestinal tract—a severe lack of collagen can lead to bowel ulcers, reflux, and colonic lesions.

- It is an essential element of wound healing and is even used in wound dressing to aid healing.
- It provides a protective lining for our internal organs, and lack of collagen causes damage to our organs, especially the kidneys.
- It is a major component of bone, and loss of collagen has been shown to weaken bone strength. Poor collagen quality is actually associated with osteoporosis.

Pretty impressive for a fibrous protein. We can think of collagen as a long, strong, flexible fiber, like a rope. It has a double-helix shape similar to that of DNA, but it is incredibly strong. In fact, collagen has higher tensile strength than steel!

You may be wondering what this amazing protein is made of. The components of collagen are the amino acids glycine, proline, and hydroxyproline. These are the conditionally essential amino acids discussed previously that are lacking in our diets, but that are abundant in bone broth.

Bone broth is rich in these amino acids because it literally contains the broken-down collagen of the animal. Muscle meat itself (e.g., chicken breast) is not rich in these amino acids because it does not contain a significant amount of collagen-containing connective tissue. In fact, we usually intentionally remove any connective tissue, or "gristle," that happens to make its way to our plate. By consuming bone broth, we add the missing pieces—these amino acids that serve as the literal building blocks of our body.

This answers a very common question that I hear about bone broth, even from healthcare professionals, which goes something like, "How can the collagen in bone broth be helpful when the molecule is too large to be absorbed?" The answer is that collagen is broken down into these conditionally essential amino acids, which are absorbed and then used to re-create collagen. Indeed, supplementation with collagen has been shown to be beneficial in a variety of situations:

- Collagen improves rating scores for joint pain and tenderness in people with osteoarthritis.
- Collagen has been shown by several studies to improve rheumatoid arthritis symptoms better than placebo. It even performed nearly as well as the medication Methotrexate but without the common side effects of that

medication (which include bleeding, stomach pain, inflammation, diarrhea, sepsis, feeling dizzy, and/or vomiting).

- Collagen can be used to increase tissue growth of bones, blood vessels, and wounded tissue. On the other hand, lack of collagen is associated with osteoporosis.

Another place where collagen shows up is in the ingredient lists of beauty products. Unfortunately, collagen cannot be absorbed through the skin. Cellulite provides an example of this. Cellulite occurs when the collagen-containing connective tissue of the skin weakens. This allows fat tissue to literally bulge out between the fibers of the connective tissue. Using collagen creams on cellulite does nothing to improve it. Similarly, injectable collagen for wrinkles has temporary effects. Collagen must be produced internally for it to serve its function. The best way to use collagen to firm the skin, decrease wrinkles, and lessen cellulite is to consume it in bone broth.

Speaking of creams and supplements, it is important to note that there are actually many forms of collagen—sixteen, to be exact. The different types are found in different areas of the body. For example, type I is found in the skin. Type II collagen is found in the cartilage of joints. Supplements often contain only one type of collagen and are quite expensive. On the other hand, bone broth made from real animals contains a large variety of types and is very inexpensive per serving. Thus, I recommend including skin, cartilage, marrow, and bone in your broth whenever possible.

It is also important to consider that vitamin C is essential for the creation of collagen. Many people in the Western world underconsume vitamin C. On the other hand, ancestral diets contain an abundance of vitamin C in the forms of citrus, berries, cruciferous vegetables, and leafy greens.

There are also some key factors that can degrade collagen production. These include smoking and chronically elevated blood glucose. We all know someone who has a long smoking history and poor skin quality. This is only one visible sign of the systemic collagen breakdown that smoking causes.

With regard to blood glucose, studies have found that patients with diabetes actually have increased amounts of glycosylated collagen. This means that a sugar molecule has been added to collagen, and this weakens it, decreasing its function. This effect is the major reason why diabetes is associated with coronary artery disease and osteoporosis—the tissues are weakened by the glycosylation of collagen.

Again, this brings us back to ancestral diet and lifestyle. Smoking obviously isn't an ancestral habit. Also, ancestral diets greatly lower blood glucose levels and can even improve type II diabetes as described earlier. Thus, bone broth combined with an ancestral diet and lifestyle is the ideal way to improve collagen status.

Cartilage

Cartilage is the final beneficial component of bone broth that we should understand. Cartilage really brings together the other beneficial components that we've already discussed. It is a tissue composed of collagen (that is made of the amino acids glycine and proline), proteoglycans (remember chondroitin, glucosamine, and hyaluronic acid), and water.

Cartilage is the tissue that forms the structure of our esophagus, ears, and nose. It also lines and protects the ends of bones (hyaline cartilage). A loss of hyaline cartilage is the cause of osteoarthritis. Because cartilage has no blood vessels within it, it is slow to heal and regenerate.

Just as with collagen, cartilage cannot be simply absorbed by our gut in whole form. The process of making bone broth breaks down animal cartilage, and it is further broken down by our own digestion. The individual components are then absorbed and used to generate our own cartilage.

Contrary to popular belief, new cartilage *can* be generated, and oral supplementation of cartilage stimulates this new growth. Dr. John Prudden produced a large body of research on cartilage, finding that collagen powder supplementation greatly improved collagen synthesis in wound healing. His research found that cartilage supplements not only increased cartilage formation, but they also increased the number of fibroblasts, the cells that create and maintain cartilage.

Another fascinating finding of Dr. Prudden's research was that cartilage is a cancer-fighting compound. He found that cartilage has potent anti-inflammatory and immunoregulatory capabilities. His human trials with bovine cartilage eliminated at least 70 percent of myeloma and ovarian, pancreatic, colon, testicular, and sarcoma tumor cells. Dr. Prudden also found in a human trial that 90 percent of cancer patients responded to cartilage supplementation. Improvement was seen in a wide variety of cancers: pancreas, lung, ovary, rectum, prostate, cervix, and thyroid. However, it is important to note that Dr. Prudden used bovine cartilage over a period of years to yield these results. Recent studies have looked at the effectiveness of shark cartilage to improve cancer and found no effect. However, these treatment courses did not occur over a period of years, and shark cartilage may have different properties than that of cows.

There is no clinical trial to conclusively say how cartilage fits into cancer- or any other treatment, but I agree with the stance of the Weston A. Price Foundation: Bone broth should be taken at a dose of one cup (8 ounces) per day for prevention on an ongoing basis, and of three cups (24 ounces) per day when seeking clinical improvement for a disease or condition.

3

Bone Broth Healing Powers

If you look online for information about the benefits of bone broth, you can find some pretty outlandish claims. I've seen confident statements that it will cure specific diseases and conditions. These claims are usually not backed up with references, or I often see these articles citing each other. It's like an endless game of telephone.

My honest opinion is that, while these articles obviously mean to encourage intake of this healthful food, they actually undermine its credibility. I don't see a lot of healthcare professionals recommending bone broth. In my opinion, part of the reason is that bone broth is not always discussed in a responsible way. So, my goal with this book is to provide you with the real evidence regarding bone broth: what's actually there and what isn't.

Truth be told, there are no human clinical trials studying the effects of bone broth. The best we have is evidence for the individual components of bone broth. We also have the ancestral history of bone broth to help guide us. Bone broth is an ancient food which humans have been consuming for a large part of our history. This fact improves our confidence that bone broth should be a part of our diet.

We also don't have evidence to show what "dose" of bone broth should be used. Some studies showing benefits of the components of bone broth have used higher doses of those components than bone broth would normally provide. However, keep in mind that many of the components of bone broth are under-consumed in a "normal" diet. Thus, some bone broth is better than none. When we drink bone broth *and* adopt an ancestral diet, we get even closer to consuming what our bodies need (and less of what it doesn't).

So, in this book and with my clients, I start with the Weston A. Price Foundation's recommendation of one cup of bone broth daily for wellness and three cups daily for healing. I also recommend an ancestral diet and lifestyle in conjunction with bone broth, to the degree that it is possible and practical. I describe exactly what that means in future chapters. The twenty-one day duration of this program is an ideal way to test how you feel with these changes. If you find that they benefit you, I provide more details later in the book outlining how to proceed after the twenty-one days.

As for individual diseases and conditions, I will briefly summarize the evidence that supports the use of bone broth. Any of these topics could be a book of their own, so please don't take this as a complete discussion of the topic. I aim to simply introduce the disease or condition, then to show how bone broth fits in.

Also, please keep in mind that for any disease or condition you should first get care from a healthcare professional. Discuss with them the use of bone broth as a part of your treatment plan. I find that it is generally safe to recommend bone broth as it is unlikely to cause problems in most situations. However, there are cases where it is prudent to be careful. Examples of when caution is warranted with bone broth include histamine intolerance and food sensitivities to any of the ingredients (including glutamine). Both histamine intolerance and food sensitivities produce a large variety of symptoms, so if you have trouble with bone broth or suspect that you might, I recommend getting advice from a healthcare professional experienced in these areas.

Keep in mind that some conditions do require additional dietary changes beyond bone broth and the "baseline" ancestral diet. Therapeutic diets such as low-FODMAP, autoimmune paleo, Specific-Carbohydrate Diet (SCD), Gut and Psychology Syndrome (GAPS), low-histamine, anti-candida, gluten-free, etc. should be implemented and monitored with the help of a trained professional. If you wish to find a functional, integrative, ancestral physician and/or dietitian, I have provided some ways to get started in the Resources section on page 192.

Joint Health:
Osteoarthritis and Rheumatoid Arthritis

The compounds in bone broth have been extensively studied for joint health, and there is good evidence that they provide benefits. Osteoarthritis is the weakening and damage of the tissue between articulating bones and the surrounding/supporting joints. It results in pain and limited range of motion. Bone broth provides the building blocks needed to repair the cartilage and synovial fluid of the joint. Studies have found that glycine, glucosamine, chondroitin, hyaluronic acid, N-acetylgalactosamine, and collagen all provide improvement of osteoarthritis symptoms. Bone broth provides all of those compounds in real-food form.

Whereas osteoarthritis is the mechanical breakdown and damage of a joint, rheumatoid arthritis is an autoimmune condition in which the immune system attacks the joint tissues. The resulting inflammation and damage causes pain, swelling/stiffness, and decreased range of motion. As described above, bone broth provides the often-lacking dietary components required to re-build joint tissue.

However, when it comes to autoimmune disease, bone broth provides additional benefits. Many of its compounds are anti-inflammatory and immune-modulating—two crucial factors in management of autoimmune disease. All of the conditionally essential amino acids in bone broth are known to support proper immune function. Remember also that chicken bone broth has been shown to improve immunity. The amino acids and glycoproteins in bone broth are essential in the body's anti-inflammatory pathways, such as for the production of the master antioxidant glutathione. The specific components of bone broth that have been shown to improve Rheumatoid Arthritis symptoms are glucosamine, N-acetylgalactosamine, and collagen.

A final way that bone broth may benefit autoimmune disease is by improving gut integrity. Poor gut lining integrity ("leaky gut") and imbalance of the microbiome (or "dysbiosis") are believed to be major contributors to autoimmune disease. These gut problems are thought to put the immune system in "overdrive," stimulating it to erroneously attack the body's own tissues. The compounds in bone broth have been shown to support gut lining integrity in several ways. Remember that glutamine has been shown to actually repair and maintain gut barrier function. Conversely, lack of dietary glutamine greatly hinders the growth of the intestinal epithelial cells. Another compound in bone broth, glucosamine, aids the production of gut-protecting mucous lining. Finally, N-acetylgalactosamine improves the blood flow and protective lining of the gastrointestinal tract. Thus, bone broth provides compounds that support gut integrity, a major factor in autoimmune disease.

To me, bone broth for either type of arthritis is a no-brainer. It is important to remember, though, that arthritis studies showing benefits from these compounds suggest that several months of treatment are required to see results. This is especially true for the repair of slow-growing cartilage tissue.

Athletic Performance

There are two primary reasons why I recommend bone broth for athletes. The first is that joints take a beating in most kinds of sports/exercise. As described above, bone broth provides the nutrients needed for joint repair, and these nutrients are not usually consumed in sufficient quantities in the typical diet. In fact, lack of these nutrients is known to be more pronounced when demand is high—such as when they are required for healing and exercise recovery. Thus, bone broth is an excellent way to support joint health and healing in the athlete.

The second reason why I recommend bone broth to athletes is for its ability to support anti-inflammatory pathways. Although exercise is a healthy habit in most cases, it does create tissue damage and inflammation. This inflammation is a healthy response to exercise; it allows the healing process to occur. However, many modern humans live in a chronically inflamed state due to our diet and lifestyle choices. Our inflammation-resolving antioxidant pathways such as glutathione are pretty tapped out. In order to properly recover from exercise, we need the ability to resolve inflammation. Bone broth can provide the support to do just that.

Strong Hair, Skin, Teeth, and Nails

It's a sad truth, but collagen decreases with age. It is also weakened by smoking and poor blood glucose control, as discussed in Chapter 2. A lesser-known fact is that collagen is composed of the exact same conditionally essential amino acids that bone broth provides: glycine and proline. The best sources of these amino acids are animal products such as bone broth, gelatin, skin, and cured meats. When we severely limit animal protein in our diet, we also limit our ability to grow strong hair, teeth, and nails.

Scientists have actually studied the effects of collagen and found that decreased collagen is associated with wrinkles and cellulite. The integrity of our skin comes from collagen. Cellulite is literally caused by the bulging of fat tissue between weakened collagen fibers. Wrinkles are the breakdown of the collagen-based structure of our skin.

Our modern diets are lacking in the precursors needed for collagen and in the vitamin C needed to form it. To add insult to injury, our lifestyles can be harmful to the collagen we do have. Thus, although collagen does decrease with age, we further decrease it when we don't support its formation. Keep in mind that collagen can only help from the inside-out. Creams and lotions are not absorbed through the hair or skin. However, the broken-down components of collagen in bone broth *can* be absorbed by the GI tract, providing the building blocks needed for collagen. Studies have actually shown that new collagen can be created by providing the nutrients it requires. Thus, bone broth provides an excellent way to beautify from the inside-out. If you are drinking bone broth with the goal of increasing collagen, then I recommend also increasing intake of vitamin C sources such as citrus fruit, bell peppers, kiwi, broccoli, and strawberries.

Weight Loss

There are a few reasons why bone broth is a great addition to a weight loss plan, and some are more obvious than others. Of course, bone broth is a low-calorie food. Thus, it also has a low glycemic response (does not stimulate insulin release). When insulin is elevated, it signals the body to store energy as fat. Conversely, low insulin allows the opposing hormone, glucagon, to stimulate the release of triglycerides from fat tissue to be used for energy. I am not in favor of low-carbohydrate diets for most people, but I do feel that a well-designed ancestral diet is less insulin-stimulating than a "normal" Western diet and that this lower glycemic load is an extremely helpful thing—for weight loss and for health in general.

Another reason why bone broth is helpful is that it is satiating. It's kind of like getting a bang for no buck. You're getting satisfied without many calories. There is *much* more to weight loss than "calories in versus calories out." However, calories do matter to some degree in the end. Many low-calorie "diet" foods really fail to deliver in the satisfaction department. Have you ever had a 100-calorie snack pack of cookies or pretzels, only to immediately want another one . . . or two? Those kinds of foods are high in acellular carbohydrates, or refined grains. I'll go over that concept in more detail later, but for now, I'll just say that those kinds of foods are *not* satisfying. On the other hand, a warm mug of bone broth really does quell a snack urge and puts off hunger until it's actually meal time.

As we talked about, many of the compounds in bone broth are essential for health, but are lacking in modern diets. This is especially true when we are under physical stress, avoiding animal foods, or restricting our calorie intake. Bone broth is extremely low in calories. Thus, it provides a way to provide important nutrition, even while pursuing a weight loss goal.

Another interesting angle to the role of bone broth in weight loss is that it is abundant in glycine. This conditionally essential amino acid stimulates the release of human growth hormone (HGH). Two functions of HGH are to increase metabolic rate and stimulate the release of triglycerides from fat cells. It also plays a role in maintenance of bone and muscle mass. HGH is naturally released by the pituitary gland in the brain. Although it stimulates growth in children, adults continue to release HGH to a lesser degree, especially during sleep and exercise. With the exception of certain medical conditions, taking oral or injectable forms of HGH can be harmful. However, gently encouraging HGH release with glycine is not risky. In fact, it could increase metabolic rate and the release of triglycerides from fat tissue. Bone broth provides a way to provide glycine from a clean and healthful source.

The final way that bone broth supports weight loss is by benefiting gut health. The microbiome (the composition of our gut bacteria) is closely linked to weight. In fact, multiple studies have shown that obese mice who receive the gut bacteria of lean mice actually become lean and vice versa. However, this direct effect of the microbiome on weight has not been proven in humans.

Research on the microbiome is so new that we do not yet know exactly what kind of microbiome changes will aid weight loss or how exactly to create those changes. As an example of the complexity surrounding this issue, lean adults in the Western world tend to have an abundance of a family of bacteria called Bacteroidetes as opposed to another family called Firmicutes. However, hunter-gatherer tribes such as the Hadza of Tanzania are lean and incredibly healthy . . . with an abundance of Fermicutes as opposed to Bacteroidetes—just the opposite of lean Westerners. Thus, there is not solid evidence to tell you exactly how to optimize your microbiome for weight loss. However, it is clear that gut health plays a role in body weight, and that decreased microbiome diversity is correlated with obesity. Bone broth supports gut health and the microbiome by providing the precursors needed for the replacement of gut enterocytes (gut lining cells), the release of gut-protecting mucin, and the actual reparation of gut wall integrity.

Autoimmune Disease

Most people know that cardiovascular disease and cancer are two leading causes of death in the Western world. However, few realize that autoimmune disease is also a major contributor. Autoimmunity is one of the top ten leading causes of death for women under age 65. Autoimmune disease is also among the top three causes of chronic illness and disability among women in the United States. Approximately 8 percent of the United States population now has an autoimmune disease, and it is increasing at the alarming rate of 12 to 15 percent annually.

Autoimmune disease is characterized by an immune system that attacks and damages the body's own tissues. There are over 80 different autoimmune diseases such as celiac disease, multiple sclerosis, Hashimoto's thyroiditis, type I diabetes, inflammatory bowel disease (ulcerative colitis and Crohn's disease), lupus, scleroderma, psoriasis, rheumatoid arthritis, and Sjögren's syndrome.

Treatment plans for autoimmune disease depend on the specific disease and the individual, but two important areas to consider are dietary quality and gut permeability. With regard to diet, an anti-inflammatory ancestral diet is the best bet. The autoimmune paleo diet is one popular choice, and another great option is the Wahls Protocol diet. It was created by Dr. Terry Wahls, who was able to reverse her crippling multiple sclerosis using the protocol.

Part of the reason why these nutrient-dense diets may be helpful is that nutrient deficiencies contribute to autoimmunity. Two examples of this are zinc and vitamin D, both of which are important nutrients that help regulate and support the immune system yet are lacking in modern diets. In fact, the rate of autoimmunity is higher at northern latitudes; for some autoimmune diseases, the rate is even 10 times higher in northern countries than in the tropics. This fact is attributed to a lack of vitamin D in northern climates.

When it comes to gut permeability, remember from the discussion of rheumatoid arthritis that increased gut permeability is believed to be a major contributor to autoimmune disease. When the tight junctions between the cells lining the intestine are too "leaky," the immune system is exposed to foreign proteins that put it into overdrive and cause it to attack the body's own tissues. Some things that can increase gut permeability are inflammation, NSAID medications, antibiotics, high alcohol intake, stress, environmental toxins, small-intestinal bacterial overgrowth, and gut dysbiosis, in which diet plays a major role. The protein zonulin specifically modulates the tight junctions between the cells of the digestive tract, and zonulin is upregulated by the proteins in gluten. Thus, a gluten-free diet is often a part of treatment for any autoimmune disease, not just celiac.

As previously discussed, bone broth provides nutrients that are important for decreasing inflammation and that help to "heal and seal" the gut. Glutamine has specifically been shown to improve gut barrier function, and lack of glutamine hampers replacement of the short-lived cells that line the gut. Glucosamine supports production of the protective mucous that lines healthy gut tissue. N-acetylgalactosamine has also specifically been shown to improve the protective lining of the gut. Additionally, N-acetylgalactosamine decreases neurological autoimmunity and is now being studied as a therapeutic approach to multiple sclerosis.

Autoimmunity is incredibly complex and admittedly not fully understood. However, ancestral diets and bone broth are both worth implementing because they can improve nutrient deficiencies, reduce chronic inflammation, and lessen gut permeability.

Digestive Disorders

As with all of these diseases and conditions, we're only going to be able to brush the surface here. Digestive disorders are another "epidemic" in the modern world, with almost all types increasing in incidence. An astonishing 20 percent of American adults now exhibit the most common digestive disorder, Irritable Bowel Syndrome (IBS). Some other digestive disorders include IBD (ulcerative colitis and Crohn's disease), gastroparesis (slowed stomach emptying), reflux or GERD, ulcers, malabsorption, and chronic pancreatitis.

Some of the signs and symptoms of digestive disorders are the obvious diarrhea, constipation, pain, bloating, gas, and belching. However, these disorders also can have systemic effects that produce things like fatigue, poor sleep, anxiety, depression, joint and/or muscle pain, protein and/or nutrient deficiencies, and allergic symptoms. As described previously, what's often happening here is increased gut permeability. It allows proteins from our intestine to encounter the blood and immune system to a harmful degree. The result is an overactive immune system and systemic inflammation.

Fortunately, the amino acids and proteoglycans in bone broth can help heal and seal the gut. They also can help restore the mucous barrier that protects our gut lining *and* feeds the beneficial gut bacteria who live there. The amino acid glycine enhances gastric acid secretion—a good thing since stomach acid is actually often *lacking* in digestive conditions such as reflux or GERD. The proteoglycan component N-acetylgalactosamine has actually been found to improve Crohn's disease in children.

Remember that these amino acids and proteoglycans are the broken-down components of the cartilage and collagen in our broth. Cartilage specifically was shown by the research of Dr. Prudden to successfully treat ulcerative colitis and Crohn's disease. A lack of collagen can cause bowel ulcers, reflux, and colonic lesions.

Despite these benefits, there is some controversy regarding the use of bone broth for specific digestive conditions. One is small-intestinal bacterial overgrowth (SIBO), a common cause of IBS. The other is candidiasis, fungal infection of the digestive tract. The idea here is that, because the amino acids in bone broth serve as fuel for cells, they may also fuel the bacteria or fungus that are problematic. This is an issue that I address on an individual basis with my clients, and my clinical experience has been that bone broth can actually aid treatment in many of these cases.

Overall, bone broth can help with digestive conditions in a variety of ways. It supports protection and healing of the gut. It stimulates release of stomach acid that aids digestion and prevents harmful bacteria and fungus. It supports healthy immune function, which is especially important with regard to autoimmune diseases (IBD). It helps to ease chronic inflammation and to eliminate the common underlying cause ("leaky gut"). Thus, bone broth is almost always useful for addressing digestive conditions.

Osteoporosis

Osteoporosis is incredibly common, and a calcium supplement is not helpful for avoiding it. In modern society, women have a 50 percent chance of experiencing a fracture due to osteoporosis after the age of 50. For men, the chance is around one in four. The ramifications of this are large; even minor bone fractures due to osteoporosis significantly increase risk of mortality.

Most people are surprised to learn that the United States has one of the highest rates of osteoporosis in the world *and* among the highest intakes of calcium in the world. Systemic review of the literature has found that supplemental calcium really does *not* decrease fracture risk, and that it can actually *increase* risk of cardiovascular disease and kidney stones.

So, the answer to osteoporosis is not simply calcium. Two additional nutrients that are needed to properly utilize calcium and maintain bone health are vitamin D and K2. Both are usually lacking in modern diets but are abundant in ancestral diets.

Another major player in bone health is collagen. It is a major component of bone, and loss of collagen degrades bone strength. Poor collagen quality is actually associated with osteoporosis. Keep in mind that collagen is damaged by poor blood glucose control and smoking. This fact helps to explain why both diabetes and smoking are risk factors for osteoporosis. As we now know, bone broth is a rich source of clean, complete collagen. Thus, bone broth is a helpful food for bone health and osteoporosis because of collagen, not calcium.

Cancer

Did you know that there are two major theories as to what causes cancer? The first you have probably heard in some form: that genetic mutations allow cells to grow uncontrollably (becoming cancer cells). The second theory is actually the *original* theory that went out of favor, but it is now regaining popularity. This is the metabolic theory of cancer—that before genetic mutations take hold, there is *first* a metabolic problem. Specifically, mitochondria (the cell's energy factories) fail to produce sufficient energy, and this allows cancer cells to proliferate by use of anaerobic metabolic pathways.

The specifics are beyond the scope of this book, but keep in mind that overall cancer incidence is increasing, despite the incredible amount of funding that cancer research receives. One likely reason for this poor result is that cancer research is focused almost exclusively on the genetic theory of cancer and very little on the metabolic theory of cancer.

So, the best approach for now is to focus on the traditional cancer-prevention strategies (reducing oxidative stress, avoiding environmental toxins, and supporting healthy immunity) while also supporting the mitochondria. I don't see these as mutually exclusive at all. In fact, bone broth and ancestral diets actually do all of those things.

One of the specific ways that bone broth plays a role in cancer prevention is by providing glycine and glutamine. Remember that dietary intake of these amino acids often falls below needs. Both are required for the production of the antioxidant glutathione. Thus, the amino acids in bone broth reduce oxidative stress—a major threat to mitochondria and a known cancer risk factor. Another feature of glutamine is that it stimulates the tumor-suppressing gene p53. Activation of p53 is known to cause the death (apoptosis) of cancer cells. Although glutamine can serve as fuel for cancer cells, it also fuels and supports the immune cells that are critically needed to combat cancer. Thus, I don't support the idea that glutamine avoidance is necessary in cancer treatment plans—in fact, glutamine helps to fight cancer cells.

The proteoglycans in bone broth also play a role against cancer. The combination of glucosamine and chondroitin reduces C-reactive protein (CRP), a marker of inflammation. Their long-term use is associated with lower risk of colorectal and lung cancer. There is also a connection between breast cancer and problems with N-acetylgalactosamine.

Also, remember that long-term use of bovine cartilage was shown to eliminate at least 70 percent of myeloma and ovarian, pancreatic, colon, testicular, and sarcoma tumor cells. In this human trial, 90 percent of cancer patients responded to cartilage supplementation. Improvement was seen in a wide variety of cancers: pancreas, lung, ovary, rectum, prostate, cervix, and thyroid.

Although even the experts don't agree as to what causes cancer, we can play an active role in preventing and treating it. Cancer is much more than simply a genetic mutation that we can't prevent. There are lifestyle and dietary factors that play major roles. Ancestral diet, lifestyle, and certainly bone broth are all wise choices with regard to cancer prevention. If you are currently undergoing cancer treatment, then please discuss any dietary or other changes with your healthcare provider.

Infections, Fibromyalgia, and Chronic Fatigue Syndrome

Bone broth and its components are incredibly supportive of immune function, which explains chicken's soup historic status as a cold or flu treatment. As described before, scientists actually studied this theory and found that it was true. Aside from acute infection, the immune-modulating function of bone broth also contributes to its beneficial role in cancer, digestive disorders, and autoimmune disease. Another area in which bone broth and immune function may play a role is chronic infection.

You may not have heard much about "chronic infection," but you probably have heard of Lyme disease, herpes simplex, and Epstein-Barr virus (the most common cause of mononucleosis, or "mono"). After the acute period of these infections, they usually persist in the body, often causing chronic symptoms. These chronic infections are believed to be major underlying causes of fibromyalgia and chronic fatigue syndrome (or systemic exertion intolerance disease). Unfortunately, it is not uncommon for the debilitating pain and fatigue of these conditions to go undiagnosed as an infection. They remain one of the most frustrating and "untreatable" conditions in modern medicine.

There is no medication that can eliminate a chronic viral infection, and although Lyme disease is bacterial, it is also incredibly difficult to treat. Thus, the answer is to fight these chronic infections from the inside-out. As described in previous sections, bone broth powerfully strengthens the immune system. As an additional benefit, bone broth helps to remedy the gut permeability and inflammation associated with both fibromyalgia and chronic fatigue syndrome. Thus, bone broth is an excellent choice for these syndromes.

Mental Health

One of the most fascinating things about the microbiome is the gut-brain connection. Studies have found that short-chain fatty acids produced by gut bacteria actually travel to the brain and decrease permeability of the blood-brain barrier. Conversely, food allergies or sensitivities, medications, exercise, mast cell activation, and stress can all release inflammatory cytokines which increase permeability of the gut *and* of the blood-brain barrier.

This increased permeability of the blood-brain barrier has been coined "leaky brain" and is associated with anxiety and depression. Thus, the protective effect of the microbiota against "leaky brain" is extremely important. Studies have actually shown that nurturing a healthy microbiome with prebiotics decreases depression and anxiety. The microbiome even has an effect on motivation, emotions, and higher cognitive functions such as intuitive decision-making. Women who eat probiotics (beneficial gut bacteria) actually have different brain responses to emotional stimuli than women who don't.

Conversely, mice without a microbiome (germ-free mice) usually demonstrate anxious and anti-social behavior. When gut bacteria are transferred from a healthy mouse to a germ-free one, the normal *behavior* of the healthy mouse actually transfers with it.

So, the gut-brain connection is pretty powerful. This brings us back to bone broth. Bone broth nurtures a healthy microbiome by providing the often-lacking amino acids it needs. Bone broth also supports production of the mucous that our microbiome uses for fuel. Normally the microbiome uses dietary fiber as its fuel source, but dietary fiber is severely limited in most diets. Adults in modern societies consume around 10 grams per day (less than half of the recommendation), as opposed to hunter-gatherers who consume around

100 grams per day. When fiber is absent, gut bacteria consume the mucous that should be naturally present. However, modern diets don't normally contain the nutrients needed to produce sufficient mucous for the microbiome. Thus, the modern microbiome is starving to death.

Two amino acids in bone broth have specifically been connected with mental health, and both of them are limited in modern diets. Glycine acts as an inhibitory neurotransmitter that reduces anxiety and increases calmness. Glutamine has been suggested as a "brain food" that can help improve depression, anxiety, and ADHD.

So, between our starving microbiomes and nutrient-poor diets, it is no wonder that mental health conditions are so commonplace. More than 1 in 10 Americans over the age of 12 now take antidepressant medication, although the effects of these medications are almost nonexistent except in the most severe cases. In short, pharmacology doesn't have a good answer to mental health conditions.

Bone broth supports a healthy microbiome and thus contributes to an improved gut-brain axis—a known player in depression and anxiety. It also provides the missing amino acids needed for optimal neurological function. In fact, bone broth is a cornerstone of the popular and effective GAPS diet that was designed by Dr. Campbell-McBride to address neurological and psychiatric conditions. So, for mental health, I recommend combining bone broth with an ancestral diet. This combination can support the microbiome. It also aids other root-cause players of mental health by reducing chronic inflammation and correcting nutrient deficiencies.

4

Digging Deeper:
Dietary Supplements
vs. Real Broth

It isn't always convenient to keep a big pot of bones stewing away on the back burner. Bone broth also isn't something that lends itself to research, as each batch will be slightly different, and it can't really be patented. Thus, many consumers and researchers use products that attempt to create the benefits provided by bone broth but in a more convenient fashion. Examples include collagen-enriched beauty products, MSG, gelatin, and supplements such as glucosamine and chondroitin. But how do these products compare to real broth?

The answer is: not very well. The problem is that none of these products contain the full array of bone broth's beneficial components. In the example of beauty products, collagen cannot be absorbed through the skin. Injectable collagen provides a temporary fix. The collagen is eventually absorbed by the body, and the wrinkles come right back.

As discussed previously, MSG is at best unhelpful and at worst a neurotoxin to which some people are highly reactive. Most broth, stock, canned soup, and seasoning packets contain MSG as an alternate source of the savory glutamates that real broth contains. With regard to health benefits, there is simply no comparison.

Gelatin and collagen powders are a popular supplement, and these components of bone broth are responsible for many of its benefits. Most commercial gelatin is created using animal hides, so it only contains one form of collagen—type I. On the other hand, bone broth contains the collagen from many parts: the bones themselves, the cartilage, and the skin. Thus, bone broth provides more types of collagen. In addition, commercial gelatin powders do not contain the other important components of gelatin besides collagen.

More importantly, the source of the animal is not known with commercial gelatin. In fact, we are pretty much guaranteed that the animals used to make commercial gelatin were conventionally grown. This means that they were likely fed conventional, genetically-modified grains containing the pesticide glyphosate.

As discussed previously, glyphosate (commercially known as Roundup) is derived from the amino acid glycine and actually can *replace* glycine in protein molecules. Thus, glycine-rich gelatin and collagen can be rich in glyphosate, a pesticide implicated in cancer, autoimmune disease, neurological disease, and autism. So, although gelatin and collagen powders can be helpful, quality sourcing is key. Just as with bones for broth, gelatin and collagen powders should come from organic, grass-fed sources only.

Another popular dietary supplement is glucosamine and chondroitin. As discussed before, these are important proteoglycan/GAGs (the side chains) found in bone broth, and they have been shown by research studies to provide significant benefits. However, just as with gelatin, these supplements fall short of providing the full complement of beneficial compounds that bone broth contains.

More importantly, use of dietary supplements introduces a whole new element of risk. I use dietary supplements frequently in my practice, so I am NOT against them. However, it is important to know that dietary supplements are not regulated by the United States Food and Drug Administration (FDA) like medications. They are regulated much more like foods. Thus, they are not tightly controlled or tested. As a result, dietary supplements commonly contain either contaminants, less ingredients than claimed, none of the claimed ingredient, or ingredients that were not declared on the label! Dietary supplements also often contain the inexpensive forms of nutrients that are not easily converted to the active form needed by the body.

There *are* professional lines of dietary supplements that are extremely high in quality and that submit to intensive *voluntary* testing. Thus, if you do decide to take glucosamine and chondroitin or any other dietary supplement, I recommend working with a healthcare professional to source quality products from professional brands.

Lead Concerns Debunked

You may have heard of a study that came out in 2013 reporting "high" levels of lead in bone broth made with "organic" chickens. Unfortunately, I still see clients and even clinicians concerned about bone broth for this reason. In fact, the findings of the study were shown to be completely unfounded. First of all, the highest lead levels they found in broth (9.5 micrograms/liter) are well below the Environmental Protection Agency's (EPA) limits for tap water (15 micrograms/liter). So, the lead levels found in the study were not actually high. More importantly, other bone broth samples have been shown to contain no traceable levels of lead.

So, what happened? The study was thoroughly investigated by the Weston A. Price Foundation, who found that the study authors had conflicts of interest AND lived in an area where soil lead contamination is common. In fact, the study found higher lead levels in broth *with* skin rather than without. This fact indicates that the lead contamination likely came from soil lead contamination. Thus, if you source your chickens from an area without lead-contaminated soil, then your broth will not be contaminated by lead in the skin. Most shockingly, the study authors eventually admitted that the chickens used in the study were NOT, in fact, organic. They actually came from a local grocery store.

In the end, you have nothing to worry about with regard to lead in your bone broth. What this all affirms is that sourcing of your bones is important. Ensure that you are using quality, organic sources, and try to include a variety of animal types and sources. This ensures that you minimize the impact of any contaminated source.

The Importance of Sourcing

I get it. It's hard to find organic chickens and even harder to find organic, grass-fed beef bones. There is also a major cost difference. I hate to come down hard on this topic because I worry that, if the bar is too high, people won't even try. If you look around online you will find that everyone advises you to source ONLY organic, grass-fed bones. There *is* a difference. But, I'm going to let you in on a little secret. I tell my clients to just do the best they can. And they get incredible results, even with conventional bones. The reason is that our bodies are *thirsty* for these nutrients. So, if you use a conventional, grocery store animal in your broth, you're still making bone broth. If that's the best you can manage, then do it!

All that being said, there are significant differences between the two. In fact, some of my clients have even commented to me that they could taste and *smell* the difference when they used organic, grass-fed bones. I agree! They really do produce less "sludge" at the top of the broth, they taste better, and they are more healthful. One of the differences was discussed above; conventional animals contain the harmful pesticide glyphosate in their tissues, *especially* in the glycine-rich collagen.

Antibiotics are another major concern with conventional animals. It's no secret that conventionally grown animals receive a significant amount of antibiotics that they then pass on to whoever eats their meat. One major problem with this widespread antibiotic use is the increase in antibiotic-resistant bacteria. These superbugs pose significant public health risks. On an individual level, antibiotics threaten the healthful bacteria of our gut, the microbiome. The modern microbiome already struggles in a world of low fiber (its food), common antibiotic prescriptions, cesarean section deliveries, and surprisingly low levels and duration of breastfeeding. A dysfunctional microbiome is associated with a vast number of diseases, all of which are increasing in incidence. Some of these include Irritable Bowel Syndrome (IBS), autoimmune disease, neurological disease, and mental health disorders such as anxiety and depression. Thus, avoidance of additional antibiotic exposure via meat is advisable.

Another concern with regard to bone sourcing is lead. Remember from before that the study finding high levels of lead in their bone broth used conventional, grocery store–sourced chicken in an area where soil lead contamination was high. Their study even revealed that the lead contamination in their broth came from the skin of the animal—not the bones themselves. Thus, bones are not inherently high in lead, but lead-contaminated soil will increase lead levels in the skin of the animal. This lead will make its way into the broth. Thus I recommend sourcing from a variety of locations and companies if possible, so that the risk of contamination is decreased. There are also websites that offer the ability to look up lead contamination levels in specific areas. Within the United States, a good resource is the Environmental Protection Agency's Consumer Confidence Reports (https://www.epa.gov/ccr).

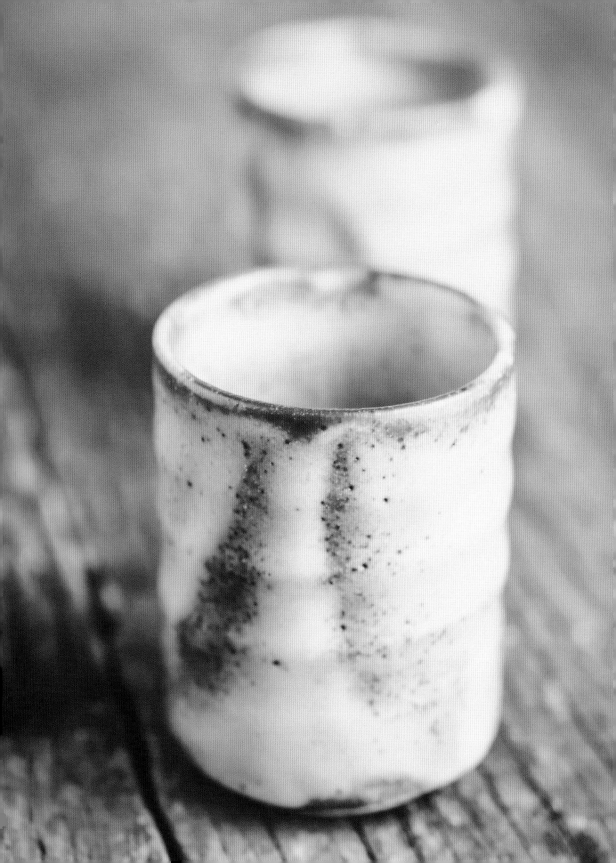

PART II

Beyond Bone Broth

Reap the Full Benefits of Bone Broth with an Ancestral Diet and Lifestyle

I hope by now you're convinced that bone broth is an important addition to your diet. While adding it will absolutely benefit you, I encourage you to take it one step further. Bone broth is just one missing piece of the traditional diets that make us thrive. So, I encourage you to combine bone broth with other ancestral foods to reap the full healing, life-changing benefits. In this section, I will explain the why and how of doing just that.

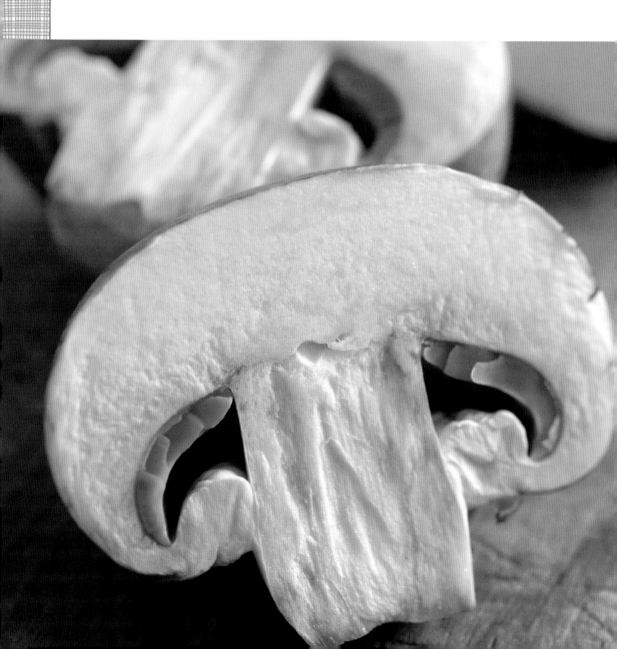

5

Ancestral Diet Overview

Herein lies the answer to *why* we are experiencing an epidemic of chronic disease in the modern world. For over 200,000 years, humans subsisted on a diet consisting mostly of meat, poultry, fish, eggs, fruit, vegetables, nuts, seeds, and herbs/spices. Although there was some variety by area with regard to this diet, there were obviously no processed foods.

Agriculture began around 10,000 years ago. The premise behind ancestral diets is that there simply has not been enough time or genetic pressure for humans to adapt to the foods that came with agriculture. Examples of these foods include grains, industrial seed and vegetable oils, soy, processed sugar, and food additives (i.e. dyes, gums, and preservatives). Dairy and legumes (beans) remain a gray area that is based on genetics, personal tolerance, and types/preparations of those foods. The human diet has changed so dramatically to these foods that we now consume at least 70 percent of our energy from foods that were never consumed by our ancestors.

The benefits of abandoning these foods in favor of ancestral ones are no less than astounding. There is NO medication or dietary supplement that comes close to providing the health benefits gained by eating the foods our bodies were designed to expect. Evidence has shown that ancestral diets:

- Improve risk factors for metabolic syndrome. Ancestral diets lower waist size, total cholesterol, LDL cholesterol, blood pressure, liver fat, and fasting blood glucose while increasing HDL. This effect is found for a wide variety of test subjects: healthy controls, obese postmenopausal women, type II diabetics, and cardiovascular disease patients.
- Improve glucose tolerance and decrease waist size more powerfully than a Mediterranean diet.
- Lower risk factors for cardiovascular disease—body weight, BMI, waist circumference, blood pressure, plasminogen activator inhibitor-1 (a marker of atherosclerosis), and CRP (a marker of inflammation).
- Improve blood glucose control and lower hemoglobin A1C in type II diabetics.

Amazingly, these impressive results were found in relatively short studies (ten days to three months in duration). So, you don't need to wait long to get remarkable benefits from an ancestral diet. Just the twenty-one day program outlined in this book will get you impressive results.

One common misperception I hear about ancestral diets is that they are almost completely meat-based. In fact, a well-balanced ancestral diet is composed of mostly plants, with a small to medium serving of meat, poultry, seafood, or eggs at most meals. Interestingly, though, hunter-gatherers did consume approximately 65 percent of their energy from animal sources and were relatively free from signs or symptoms of cardiovascular disease and diabetes. Thus, excess meat consumption is not a concern with regard to well-designed ancestral diets.

Hunter-gatherers also ate fairly high-fat diets, at least as high as is currently consumed by Western societies. The amount of dietary cholesterol they consumed was similar or even higher to that of Americans. It is important to understand, though, that dietary cholesterol has been shown *not* to have a major effect on serum cholesterol and risk of heart disease. In fact, dietary cholesterol was removed as a "nutrient of concern" by the scientific committee of the 2015 US Dietary Guidelines. Dietary cholesterol was also found not to be a risk factor for cardiovascular disease by a joint task force of the American College of Cardiology and American Heart Association. In fact, dietary fat in general (even saturated!) has been exonerated as being unhealthful when it comes from appropriate sources and is part of an overall healthful diet.

One important difference between diets then and now is that hunter-gatherers consumed much more omega-3 and less omega-6 fats than modern societies do. Omega-3 fats reduce inflammation. On the other hand, omega-6 fats (such as those found in canola, corn, or vegetable oil) promote inflammation and heart disease. It is also important to note that traditional societies consumed only game animals, which have a different fat profile than modern supermarket meat. These animals have more mono- and polyunsaturated fats and less saturated fat. They also have more omega-3 and less omega-6 fats. Hence, grass-fed and free-range meat should be consumed if at all possible.

The fat profile isn't the only difference between meat then and now. Because hunter-gatherers consumed more parts of the animal, such as from organ meats and broth, they got more nutrients from the animal foods they consumed. For example, liver is an absolute superfood that provides high amounts of nutrients not found in muscle meats. These include vitamins A and K, iron, copper, zinc, selenium, potassium, folate, and vitamin B$_{12}$. Notably, these nutrients are largely deficient in the modern American diet.

Traditional societies also consumed a much higher amount of antioxidants, fiber, vitamins, and phytochemicals from the many plants they consumed. They consumed fewer carbohydrates and no refined carbohydrates (like those in sugar or flour). High carbohydrate intake has been shown to increase risk factors for cardiovascular disease such as blood triglycerides. Hunter-gatherers also had more healthful lifestyle habits such as high exercise, more sleep, and lack of smoking.

Thus, although it requires meat consumption, an ancestral diet and lifestyle does not increase risk of heart disease. In fact, it was shown in several human studies to lower the risk factors of both heart disease and diabetes.

Another important feature of ancestral diets is that they support a healthy gut microbiota and thus reduce risk of many modern chronic diseases. For example, obesity has been shown to be greatly caused by a combination of leptin resistance (the body stops reading the signal to stop eating) and obesogenic signaling of the gut microbiome.

Note that obesity is NOT significantly linked to a specific macronutrient balance. Review articles show that weight loss results are fairly similar between low-carbohydrate or low-fat diets. Further, traditional societies remain lean with an incredible range of carbohydrate intake—from mostly carbohydrates near the equator to nearly no carbohydrates among northern Inuit tribes. So, the common thread among traditional societies is not their macronutrient intake. The commonality is that they consume cellular carbohydrate sources rather than acellular ones.

Cellular carbohydrates are simply the carbohydrate sources that come from plants, such as root vegetables, cruciferous vegetables, and fruit. These cellular carbohydrates have lower carbohydrate density and high amounts of fiber. This allows them to nourish an anti-inflammatory, properly signaling gut microbiome. This healthy gut microbiome does a lot more than help us avoid obesity. The microbiome has been linked with cancer, autism, autoimmune disease, anxiety, depression, and neurological disease. Want to avoid these diseases? Focusing on cellular carbohydrates is the place to begin.

On the other hand, acellular carbohydrates include grains, flour, and sugar. Yes, that includes whole grains. These carbohydrate foods promote inflammation and fail to nurture our gut microbiome. In fact, they are digested well before reaching the large intestine; consuming them literally starves our gut microbiome. They also promote leptin resistance, which further contributes to obesity. Unfortunately, acellular carbohydrates make up the *vast* majority of the carbohydrate consumption of modern societies.

As a case in point, it's not uncommon for me to have a client who tells me that they eat a healthy diet and can't understand the reason for their weight gain. I will collect a food journal and find the following:

Breakfast: Whole grain cereal (grains) with non-fat milk (milk sugar)
Snack: Protein bar (sugar and often grains)
Lunch: Turkey wrap in whole-grain tortilla (flour/grains, a *few* veggies)
Snack: Usually a processed grain such as pretzels or a granola bar
Dinner: Finally, some vegetables. And more grains.

Can you see how 80 to 90 percent of carbohydrate calories can easily come from acellular carbohydrates, even with what people think is a "healthy" diet? No wonder we keep getting less and less healthy, no matter how hard we try.

The only way back to vital health is to get back to eating the diets our bodies were designed to utilize. Ancestral diets are anti-inflammatory, nutrient-rich, nurturing of the gut microbiome, and helpful for almost all chronic diseases—diabetes, cardiovascular disease, cancer, autoimmune disease, neurological conditions, mental health, and fighting obesity.

By now, you may be wondering what you would even eat on an ancestral diet. Trust me: LOTS of things and they are DELICIOUS. Imagine how it would feel to eat fat in abundance without fear, to not feel hunger, and to eat only great-tasting food—all while losing weight and improving your health. *That* is ancestral eating in a nutshell.

As for what foods it includes, I provide a detailed table later in this book and the twenty-one day plan contains exclusively ancestral recipes. But, for now, ancestral diets include meat, seafood, poultry, eggs, nuts, seeds, fruits, vegetables, ancestral fats, spices, and herbs. They emphasize nose-to-tail eating and fermented foods. They don't include grains, processed seed or vegetable oils, soy, processed sugar, or artificial ingredients. Dairy and legumes are gray areas that need to be assessed for individual tolerance, and only specific types should be consumed. The twenty-one day plan in this book does not include dairy or legumes because I recommend starting without them, then adding carefully to test tolerance.

6

Ancestral Lifestyle

Have I convinced you yet that you should be eating like a caveman or cavewoman? If so, then why not take it a step further and consider an ancestral lifestyle? In truth, diets are only one way in which modern lifestyles differ from those of our ancestors. The agricultural revolution that resulted in the major modern dietary changes was approximately 11,000 years ago. Although that may sound like a long time, consider that it was only 366 generations ago, and 0.5 percent of human history.

Genetic adaptations to our environment occur as a result of random, advantageous mutations that increase the success of survival and reproduction. In other words, the environment creates "selective pressure" on a species, and the genetics of that species changes very gradually as a result of random, rare mutations. Because these advantageous mutations occur so rarely, genetic change occurs *very* slowly; for humans, it has not occurred to any large degree in that small 0.5 percent of human history since our diets changed.

The one exception is the gene for digestion of lactose. In some cultures that have a long history of dairy consumption, they have gained the genetic ability to digest lactose as adults. These populations were northwestern Europeans and some sub-Saharan African tribes. Now, approximately 35 percent of the world's population has the genetic ability to digest lactose as an adult.

As a parallel, consider that modern, Western lifestyles came about not during the Agricultural Revolution but during the *Industrial* Revolution. The Industrial Revolution was only seven generations ago—0.009 percent of human history! There has been virtually no time for selective pressure to create real genetic changes since then. Thus, we are fundamentally mismatched between not only our diet but our *lifestyles*.

Researchers have actually been able to measure the effects of this mismatch in real time. There are still tribes of traditional hunter-gatherers in the world. These tribal people have been found to have lower blood pressure, body mass index (BMI), waist circumference, and fasting leptin than industrialized humans.

They also have higher VO$_2$ max (a marker of fitness), better visual acuity, and better bone health. When hunter-gatherers move to modern environments, these differences begin to disappear fairly quickly: tribal people begin to lose their superior fitness, body composition, and health markers. Then, when tribal people return to their traditional environments, they return to their original healthful status. It is not our genes that have changed. It is our environment that explains our current state of poor health.

Fortunately, there are several key areas of our modern environment that are the primary contributors to poor health, and we do have some ability to improve in these areas. These key areas include: sleep, stress, exercise, and environmental toxins. Each of these topics could be (and is) an entire book of its own. I will discuss them briefly here, although my short description does not do them full justice.

Sleep

As for sleep, it probably comes as no surprise that we are chronically sleep-deprived. Nearly a third of adults get less than six hours of sleep per night, and the average is 6.4 hours. On the other hand, adults in traditional cultures are in bed for 7 to 8½ hours per night. Sleeping less than six hours per night is associated with low-grade, chronic inflammation, insulin resistance, and increased risk of cardiovascular disease, type II diabetes, and obesity.

Unfortunately, it's easier said than done to start sleeping more. As a mom, wife, and business owner, *I get it*: there just aren't enough hours in the day. However, sleep is so central to health that we really aren't doing ourselves any favors by cutting back on sleep. Especially if you are pursuing a health goal, this needs to be an area of focus. Here are a few hacks that my clients have found helpful for increasing sleep time:

- Avoid blue light for three hours before bed. It is a powerful suppressant of the sleep hormone melatonin. Many smartphones now allow you to automatically filter blue light during dark hours—check your settings. Alternately, you can wear blue light-filtering glasses or just avoid phones, tablets, and computers in the evening. Energy-efficient lighting also emits a significant amount of blue light.

- Get exercise during the day—but nothing intense in the three hours before bed.
- Avoid alcohol, especially more than one serving, in the evening.
- Try not to eat after dinner. I recommend a minimum twelve-hour fast between dinner and breakfast.
- Stop caffeine at noon.
- Calculate what time will be eight hours before you need to get up, and start getting ready for bed 30 minutes prior. (For example, if you need to wake up at 6 a.m. tomorrow, start getting ready for bed at 9:30 p.m. tonight.)
- Avoid watching TV or using phones/tablets in your bed.
- Use essential oils like lavender to help you relax at bedtime.
- Try a 10-minute meditation in the evening to help you wind down and relax.
- Create a positive sleep environment: dark, cool, comfortable, and quiet (or maybe with white noise).
- If you have sleep problems such as frequent waking, insomnia, or not feeling rested after eight-plus hours, there could be more going on. HPA axis dysfunction is a common phenomenon that can result in high evening cortisol which prevents you from feeling tired at bedtime. Sex hormone disruption is also a possibility, as well as a sleep disorder such as sleep apnea. Bottom line, if you can't get good sleep, it warrants your attention. I recommend working with a qualified healthcare provider to address it.

Chronic Stress

Another problematic feature of our modern environment is chronic stress. Our bodies are designed to react to stress with a fight-or-flight response. A stressor causes our sympathetic nervous system to release epinephrine (adrenaline), norepinephrine, and cortisol. This adrenaline rush provided our ancestors with an essential survival skill: the ability to run away or attack a predator. It can even occasionally help in the modern age, such as when we need to rush to meet a deadline or complete an assignment.

However, modern humans experience stress in a way never encountered by our species before. Instead of occasional and temporary stressful events, we experience nearly constant, unending stress. It comes in the form of financial burdens, unending emails, over-exercising, deadlines, constant competition, and social pressure to perform and achieve. Although these modern stressors don't look like a wild animal, our sympathetic nervous response still reacts with the release of stress hormones.

Unfortunately, a constant, low-grade dose of cortisol and adrenaline is not helping the matter. Chronically elevated stress has been shown to have the following harmful effects:

- Cortisol increases blood glucose and decreases insulin sensitivity. This effect has been cited as the connection between stress, type II diabetes, and obesity.
- Cortisol contributes to weight gain in three ways. It mobilizes fatty acids and stores them as abdominal fat. It increases appetite and cravings for high-calorie foods. Finally, the insulin resistance described above is associated with weight gain.
- Cortisol suppresses the immune system, which increases risk of illnesses such as cold and flu, cancer, gastrointestinal disease, food sensitivities, and autoimmunity.
- Stress inhibits the parasympathetic function of the gastrointestinal tract: when you need to fight, your body shuts down digestion. Elevated stress is associated with digestive conditions such as Irritable Bowel Syndrome and Irritable Bowel Disease.
- Stress hormones constrict blood vessels and increase blood pressure. In fact, stress is associated with increased risk of hypertension and cardiovascular disease.
- Chronic stress can eventually lead to adrenal insufficiency, or HPA axis dysfunction, in which the adrenals can no longer produce sufficient stress hormones. Some of the results are fatigue, frequent illness, exercise intolerance, slow healing, irritability, and depression.
- Chronic stress is additionally associated with infertility, thyroid disorders, depression, anxiety, dementia, chronic fatigue syndrome (or systemic exertion intolerance disease), and insomnia.

Although the effects of chronic stress are clear and significant, I find that reducing stress is *extremely* challenging for my clients. Our culture seems to encourage and even praise over-working. Many of my clients report that they feel guilty when they try to slow down and relax for even a few hours. I find that over-exercising is also often encouraged and praised. Although exercise is beneficial, too much really does put our bodies in stress overload. I see the effects of this constantly in clients who work out intensely nearly every day, restrict calories, and yet cannot lose a pound.

True recovery from chronic stress is a major undertaking, but there are some small steps that I have seen provide quick results. These include:

- Adopt a daily meditation habit, even for just ten minutes to start. There are many free apps and online videos to guide you.
- Begin a daily practice of moving meditation such as yoga or Tai Chi. Again, look online for free videos.
- Try adult coloring books in the evening.
- Keep a gratitude journal: every day, write down three things that you are thankful for, or even type it into a note on your phone or computer.
- Think of a hobby or activity that you love and that makes you feel happy—work to build in more time for that.
- Think about things in your life that make you feel unhappy, anxious, or upset. Spend some time writing out specific ways to reduce those things, or even consider getting counseling help to do so.
- Practice setting healthy boundaries, especially with coworkers, family, or friends who are adding stress to your life.
- Work to spend more time relaxing and having fun with people you enjoy.
- Consider your spiritual connection, self-acceptance, and confidence; work in these areas can be highly effective for some.
- Ancestral diets support blood sugar regulation and HPA axis function by omitting high-glycemic, non-cellular carbohydrates. Also, the amino acids glycine and glutamine in bone broth act as neurotransmitters that help modulate stress.

Exercise

Aside from modern diets, another "new" invention for humans is the chair. We aren't designed to sit in a car on the way to work, sit at a desk for eight hours, sit on our way home, and then sit in front of the TV. While tribal people have been found to be highly active, modern humans sit for approximately fourteen hours per day on average. Sitting is found to increase with educational level and is actually the highest among adults aged 18–39 years.

The consequences of sitting are pretty severe. Too much sitting is associated with increased risk of obesity, osteoporosis, cardiovascular disease, and hypertension.

Most of us are aware of this fact and many try to compensate by squeezing in a short, high-intensity workout. Unfortunately, it's not that simple. A 2010 study published in the *American Journal of Epidemiology* followed over 123,000 adults and found that those who sat more than six hours per day had up to a 40 percent increased risk of death within the next fifteen years, as opposed to those who sat less than three hours per day. This effect was true, *regardless of physical activity level*.

I'm not saying that you shouldn't exercise. Exercise can be helpful for reducing risk of cardiovascular disease, type II diabetes, obesity, cancer, mental health disorders, neurological disorders, osteoporosis, and sleep disorders—exercise is essential for health. My point is that one short period of exercise several times per week is not sufficient to overcome the harmful effects of too much inactivity.

As for types of exercise, I encourage more natural forms, or "functional movement." These include movements that requite a variety of muscle groups— think pull-ups instead of bench pressing, squats instead of leg extensions, and ring dips instead of triceps extensions. Keep in mind your stress level as well. High-intensity exercise provides unique benefits but does increase stress hormones, whereas low-intensity exercise does not.

I also encourage taking this functional movement mindset out of the gym or Crossfit box and into the rest of your life. Examples of ways to include natural movement into your life include the use of a standing or treadmill desk, walking or cycling to work/school, standing when possible during meetings, and hourly walking or standing breaks (there are apps that will remind you).

I do frequently have clients who are unable to exercise due to either injury or conditions such as arthritis or fibromyalgia. Remember that bone broth can support joint healing and decrease inflammation. I will give more complete exercise instruction later in the program, even if this is your situation. Even if you can't exercise right now, that doesn't mean you can't follow this program and get results.

Environmental Toxins

There is no doubt that the chemicals and compounds we encounter on a daily basis have an effect on our health. These toxins come from a wide variety of sources: pesticides, mold, heavy metals, body products, fragrance, cosmetics, cleaning products, cigarette smoke, household chemicals, furniture, medications, and even water. In fact, adults carry between 600 and 800 foreign chemicals in their body on average. Infants are born with around 200 foreign chemicals already in their body.

What real harm does this do? A research study published in the *Annals of Family Medicine* in 2012 found that around 20 percent of the population suffers from loss of chemical tolerance (has clinical symptoms) due to toxic burden. This effect has been coined "Toxin-Induced Loss of Tolerance" (TILT) or "Sensitivity-Related Illness" (SRI). Toxins have been shown to play a role in many diseases and conditions:

- Obesity
- Depression
- Anxiety
- Chronic fatigue
- Cancer
- Insulin sensitivity/diabetes
- Autism
- ADHD
- Allergies
- Digestive problems
- Intestinal permeability
- Autoimmune disease
- Fibromyalgia
- Migraines

If you suffer from any of these, toxins should definitely be on your radar. However, I would argue that people with full-blown disease aren't the only ones who need to think about toxins. We all are affected to some degree, although it may be sub-clinical.

For example, many conventional labs may be altered when toxic burden is high. These include decreased blood cell counts (WBC, RBC), increased liver enzymes (AST, ALT, GGT), increased inflammation (CRP), increased LDL and triglyceride blood lipids, increased insulin and fasting and two-hour post-prandial blood glucose, and increased metabolic markers of DNA damage (8-OHdG).

Although it is only one piece of the equation, food is a great place to start. As a rule, ancestral diets eliminate wheat, soy, and corn. This kills two birds with one stone. Removing these foods both improves the quality of the diet, and it removes crops that are frequently laden with pesticides. Eating organic, non-GMO produce takes it a step further. I do understand that organic produce can be expensive. A few steps you can take to make this affordable are:

- Look at the Environmental Working Group's (EWG) "Dirty Dozen" and "Clean 15" lists (https://www.ewg.org/foodnews). They'll tell you what produce has the most and least pesticides; focus on at least getting organic versions of the dirty dozen.
- Look for deals at a local farmers' market.
- See if you can get a subscription to an organic produce box (or community supported agriculture) in your area. (https://www.ams.usda.gov/local-food-directories/csas)
- Consider growing your own. Even just an herb plant on your windowsill is a start. You can find many free resources online for starting a small organic garden.

Some ancestral foods even support your body's natural detoxification pathways. These foods include:

- Bone broth
- Tea (black, green, oolong)
- Cruciferous vegetables (broccoli, greens, spouts, kale, cabbage, and others)
- Spices (turmeric, curry, rosemary—eat a variety)
- Berries
- Pomegranate
- Garlic and onion
- Citrus fruits
- Leafy greens & microgreens
- Cocoa
- Sesame (oil, seeds, sesame butter, tahini)

Another dietary step that supports detoxification is intermittent fasting. The following chapter describes this practice in more detail. The program in this book does incorporate the option to intermittently fast. I also describe how to know if intermittent fasting is a good choice for you.

Aside from diet, there are a variety of lifestyle factors that can reduce toxic exposure. These include:

- Avoid using plastic, especially for your food and water. There are now a good variety of glass containers available for food and water storage.
- Avoid BPA by checking container labels and trying not to touch receipts/tickets. Wash your hands if you do. Look for BPA-free cans.
- Scrutinize your personal care products using the EWG's Skin Deep database (http://www.ewg.org/skindeep/). Replace toxic ones with more natural options. This includes makeup, fragrance, hair, and body products.
- Consider mold exposure, especially where you live and work. Consider getting an ERMI test if you suspect mold (http://www.survivingmold.com/diagnosis/ermi-testing).
- Analyze your occupational and hobby exposures. Are you protecting yourself from toxic substances and chemicals that you may use or be exposed to?
- Household cleaners—there are many good recipes online to make your own, and many stores now carry more natural options. Dry cleaning is also a significant source.
- Get at least eight hours of sleep per night.
- Avoid grilling or charring meat. If you do grill for a special occasion, make sure to marinate the meat first.
- Decrease sources of stress as much as possible, as described above.
- Sweat more—by exercise and/or sauna (infrared may provide additional benefits).

Finally, some other factors that can contribute to toxic burden are genetic susceptibility and nutrient deficiencies. If you suspect that toxic burden is affecting your health (TILT or SRI), this program is one place to start. However, if you don't get full resolution using this book, I recommend working with a qualified healthcare professional who is experienced with environmental toxins.

7

Intermittent Fasting

Intermittent fasting (IF) is the practice of spending prolonged periods of time without eating and has been found to be a potent tool for weight loss, decreasing insulin sensitivity, and improving blood lipid profiles. IF is an ancestral practice. For example, modern-day hunter-gatherer communities such as the Hunzas of Northern Pakistan eat two meals per day—one midday and one early evening. IF has been recommended for thousands of years in a variety of cultures, even by great minds of medicine such as Hippocrates.

Scientific studies of IF have revealed a clear need for metabolic rest. This physiologic need is violated when food is consumed across a long daily window and especially when eating occurs during the night hours. If you think about it, the conventional wisdom that recommends a daily breakfast and six small daily meals goes against the ancestral pattern of eating described above.

In fact, studies have found no evidence that breakfast is essential for health or weight loss. Some studies even find the opposite to be true: that those who eat breakfast or late at night experience more disease than those who skip breakfast and stop eating early in the evening. A fourteen- to eighteen-hour daily fasting window is much more consistent with our ancestral history and does indeed show benefits in human trials.

With regard to the specific benefits of IF, six human trials have found it to be effective for weight loss. Some studies have found IF to provide the additional benefits of decreased fasting insulin, improved blood lipid profiles, and lowered inflammation markers (C-reactive protein and tumor necrosis factor-alpha). The practice has also been shown to aid the body in eliminating toxins, mostly by lipolysis (fat-breakdown) from toxin-containing adipocytes (fat cells).

Also, these studies found that less than 15 percent of study participants reported significant side effects such as irritability, hunger, and low energy. In fact, study participants experienced *improved* mood on average. They experienced less fatigue, tension, and anger, and they reported improved self-confidence and positive mood.

Mice who were fed according to IF protocols improved their blood glucose control, lipid profiles, rates of cancer, and inflammation markers—even when they did not lose weight. The mice also were highly sensitive to feeding according to their circadian rhythm. When mice were allowed to eat a calorie-restricted diet during night hours they experienced weight gain, fatty liver, increased insulin, and inflammation. They also developed leptin resistance, which means their body no longer recognized the signal to stop eating. However, when these mice ate the *same* amount of calories only during daytime (time-restricted feeding), they were protected from these negative outcomes.

There have not been many studies of these time-restricted feedings in humans, but one human trial found that a daily fasting window over eleven hours resulted in significant weight loss. A second time-restricted feeding study of humans found that eating only one daily meal decreased weight and fasting glucose while improving lipid profiles (increased HDL and decreased LDL).

The most studied form of time-restricted IF in humans is Ramadan religious fasting. During this period, Muslims consume food only during night hours, usually one meal at sundown and a second meal before sunrise. Meta-analysis of studies on Ramadan fasting have found that it results in decreased weight, improved lipid profiles, decreased fasting blood glucose, and lowered inflammation. In another form of religious fasting, members of the Church of Jesus Christ of Latter-Day Saints who routinely fast have lower body weight, fasting glucose, prevalence of diabetes, and coronary stenosis. A third religious group who routinely fasts is Seventh-Day Adventists. They have been found to live 7.3 years longer on average. They usually consume two meals per day: one midday and the second in the afternoon. This leaves a lengthy overnight fasting period of approximately sixteen to eighteen hours.

Another form of IF is alternate day fasting, where intake is either completely restricted or greatly reduced for a full day. This is done somewhere on the order of twice per week. Benefits have been seen for both alternate day fasting and time-restricted feeding, but time-restricted feeding is less difficult.

Overall, the literature shows that night eating is clearly not beneficial. Thus, an important feature of IF is to avoid night and even late-evening eating. Both types of IF provide benefits, but time-restricted feeding is the most realistic and easy to implement. Thus, the ideal template suggested by the literature may be to eat one meal midday and a second meal late afternoon or early evening.

Unfortunately, there is no large-scale clinical trial that demonstrates the ideal fasting protocol for humans. So, for now, we are going on our best clinical judgment based on the existing literature. Based on the studies that do exist, we know that fasting is not harmful, with the exception of specific contraindications. Some of these are pregnancy, breastfeeding, a history of disordered eating, low body fat, type I diabetes, hypoglycemia, and intense exercise. For those who exercise intensely, I don't recommend fasting on workout days.

There are also some people for whom IF simply doesn't work. I and other clinicians have observed that for some individuals, IF seems to actually increase fasting blood glucose and worsen blood glucose control. The reason for this is not well understood, but when we fast, cortisol must be released to create blood glucose from fat and muscle glycogen. Remember that dysregulation of cortisol or HPA axis dysfunction is fairly common in our over-stressed world. So, what is likely to be happening here is that for people who already have an imbalance of cortisol, IF can worsen the situation. Thus, a final contraindication for IF is HPA axis dysfunction or the common conditions that precipitate it (chronic stress, chronic illness, and/or over-exercising). I will go into more details on who should fast and when later in the book.

So, the IF protocol that most practitioners currently recommend is a daily (or nearly daily) fasting period of fifteen to eighteen hours. For men, I recommend the range of sixteen to eighteen hours, but I find that women tend to get better results in the neighborhood of fifteen to sixteen hours. This looks something like eating a final meal at 6 p.m., then eating again between 10 a.m. and 12 p.m. for men and between 9 a.m. and 10 a.m. for women. Remember that IF isn't right for everyone. There are contraindications, and sometimes it just doesn't feel right or benefit the individual. In those cases, it is no problem to revert back to a more regular eating pattern. For those who tolerate IF well, it provides a potent way to achieve weight loss, improved blood lipid profiles and blood glucose control, decrease risk of cancer, stimulate detoxification, and reduce inflammation. In this program, I combine IF with bone broth and an ancestral diet to create a powerful disease-fighting trifecta.

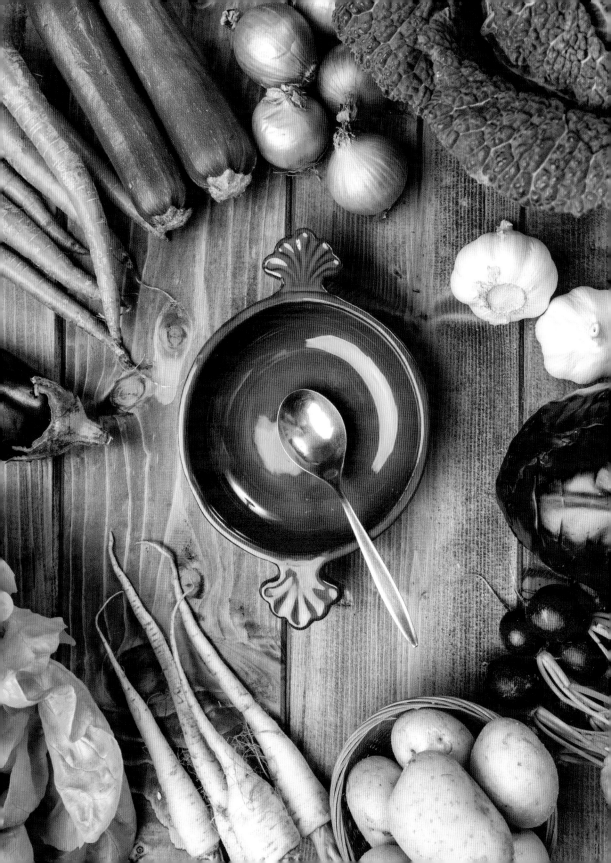

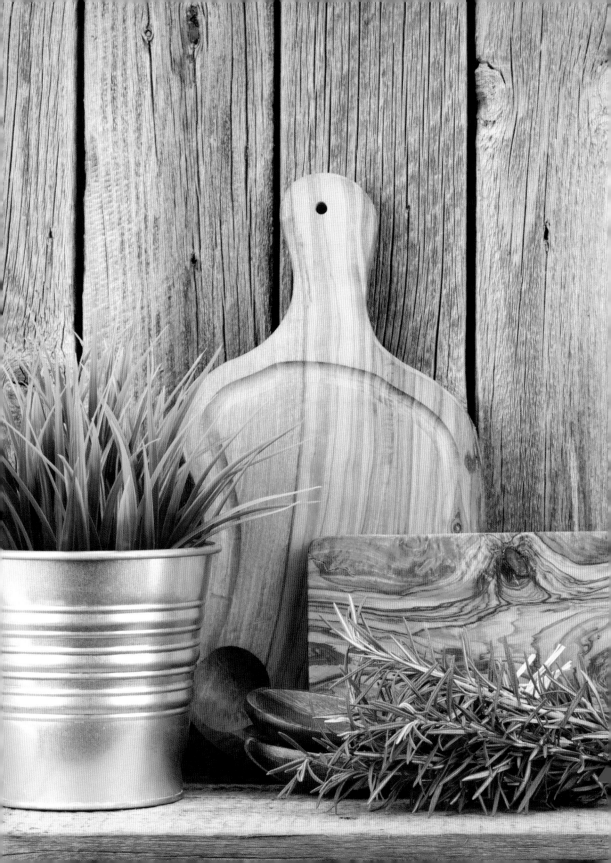

PART III

Putting It All Together

The Bone Broth Miracle Diet

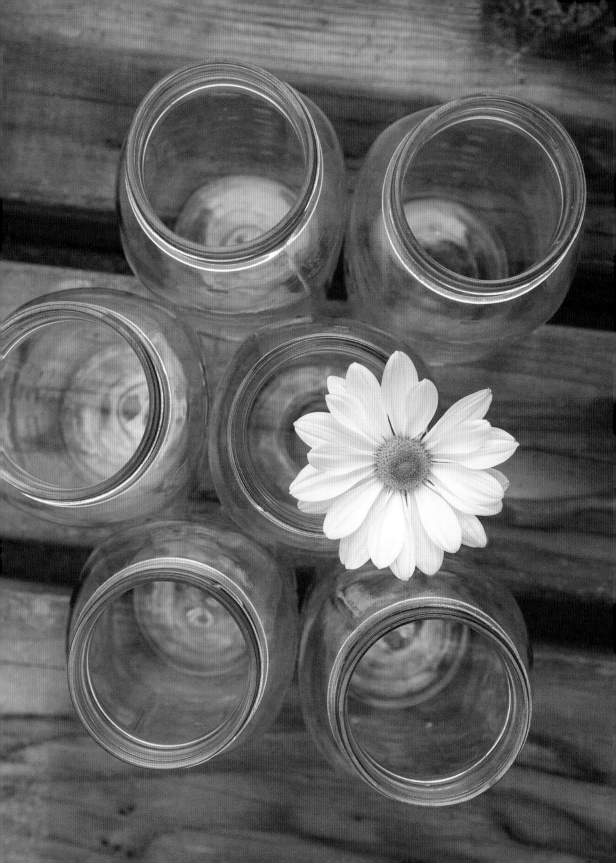

8

Getting Ready

Now that we've reviewed the principles that lay the foundation for the Bone Broth Miracle Diet, let's get started! First of all, do you have a medical condition? Don't forget to check with your healthcare provider whether this plan is appropriate for you. You can ask something like this: *"I'm planning on following a whole-foods diet from a Registered Dietitian for twenty-one days. It includes bone broth and intermittent fasting for fourteen- to eighteen-hour periods. Do you have any concerns about that?"* Examples of when bone broth could be problematic include histamine intolerance and food sensitivities to any of the ingredients.

All clear? Next you'll need to make sure you have all the equipment required:

- Mesh strainer
- Large stock pot and/or slow cooker
- Blender and/or food processor
- Chef's knife
- Cutting board
- Grater or food processor
- Large glass containers (1 quart mason jars or pop-lid preserving jars—or glass bowls work in a pinch)
- Ladle, slotted spoon, and tongs
- Dutch oven (or large stock pot)
- Food scale
- Room in your fridge/freezer (LOTS)

Got it? Ok, now let's talk bones. When it comes to bone broth, quality sources are incredibly important. You will need a source of organic (preferably free-range) chickens and grass-fed beef bones. Talk to butchers and grocers to start. Look into the Weston A. Price Foundation's resources. Look online for local farms or ranches. Ultimately, you can go online to US Wellness Meats for bones, or even purchase complete bone broth online. Check out the Resources section for more details.

Ok, got all that? Now it's time to prep for your first day! Check out the Week 1 grocery list. This list is designed for one person following the plan, so keep in mind that you will need extra for feeding a family. If you have leftovers, you can freeze them to keep the goodness going after the plan. Before you start following the plan, make sure to buy these groceries AND start your first bone broth *the day prior*. You need to hit the ground running with some broth ready to go the first morning.

Oh, and ONE more thing: the pantry clean-out. Know thyself here. If you can have ice cream sitting in your freezer and completely ignore it, then be my guest. However, if you are tempted by the food in your house, do NOT skip this step. I find that people can sometimes have pretty intense withdrawal from a "standard diet," especially from refined white flour and refined sugar. Also keep in mind that you will be fasting and may get very hungry! Is there somewhere you can send those cookies, processed snack/protein bars, leftover candy, etc.? Doing so will help support your exciting new health improvements.

9

The Bone Broth Miracle Diet

Finally, you can start! You can either follow the meal plans exclusively or design your own meals using this template. Alternately, you can do a mixture of both. If weight loss is your goal, keep reading. I'll give more details regarding specific servings sizes for weight loss later. Ideally, try to shoot for 2–3 cups of bone broth per day. With this plan you're getting two in the morning, plus sometimes extra at dinner.

- Breakfast: Have a cup of hot bone broth (salt to taste) and your morning coffee or tea. You may add a little stevia and 1 Tablespoon unsweetened almond or coconut milk to this if you want. See Fasting Tips on page 68.
- Morning snack: 150–200 calories of approved fat and/or proteins (see Ancestral Foods on page 70) and another cup of hot bone broth. Alternately, you may just drink the broth if you want to fast until lunch.
- Lunch: 4–6 ounces animal protein, 2+ cups non-starchy vegetables, a ½–1 fist-size serving of carbohydrates (fruit or starchy vegetables), and 1–2 Tablespoons ancestral fats. If you're eating fatty meat or veggies cooked in fat, that counts. Otherwise, add some.
- Afternoon snack: 150–200 calories of approved fat and/or proteins (see Ancestral Foods on page 70).
- Dinner: 4–6 ounces animal protein, 2+ cups non-starchy vegetables, a 1–2 fist-size serving of carbohydrates (starchy vegetables and maybe a little fruit), and 1–2 Tablespoons ancestral fats (already included in meat or veg counts). Try to use recipes that incorporate extra bone broth!

Tip

Fermented veggies (i.e., sauerkraut, kimchi, pickles) count toward your 2+ cups at lunch and dinner, plus you can add them to any snack. Please try to eat at least

¼ cup per day, but don't stress over it. Caution: if they're shelf stable, they're pasteurized. Go for the refrigerated section.

A Note on Alcohol

Nope, you didn't see it on the plan. Sorry. After the twenty-one days, you can experiment with wine, tequila, vodka, etc. to see how you do. That's a topic for another day. For now, I recommend stocking up on all of your favorite herbal teas. They really help out when you're craving a little something, whether it be wine or chocolate.

Fasting Tips

Yes, you read that right: we're skipping breakfast. *Gasp!* I find that there are two major camps when it comes to this: one still thinks that waking up to a big meal is essential for everyone; the second group is "all in" on the intermittent fasting game and periodically spends full days fasting.

As described earlier, scientific literature shows that intermittent fasting is extremely beneficial for insulin sensitivity, weight loss, blood lipid profile, detoxification, inflammation, and leptin resistance/appetite regulation. Interestingly, this list exactly mirrors the physiological underpinnings of the top modern diseases: heart disease, cancer, type II diabetes, obesity, and autoimmune disease. You DON'T need to go full days without eating to get the benefits.

Ideally you would eat nothing between dinner and your morning snack (other than the broth and coffee or tea). Alternately, you may extend your fast and just have broth mid-morning, skipping the morning snack. This should be a fifteen- to eighteen-hour period of time between dinner and your first snack or meal. Women should stay closer to the fifteen-hour point. Men can get away with going closer to eighteen hours if you wish.

For some people, this is no big deal. However, if you're a life-long breakfast eater like me, this could be terrifying. I LOVE breakfast. However, I have had such great results from intermittent fasting that I happily give it up for periods of time. If you think you will struggle, then here is the approach I recommend:

- Drink a big glass of water as soon as you wake up.
- Make your morning coffee or tea. You may add stevia and/or 1 Tablespoon unsweetened coconut or almond milk. Enjoy this as slowly as you can.

- Heat up your cup of broth—don't forget to add sea salt (no, salt is not bad for you). Again, try to enjoy this slowly.
- If you need to, make another coffee or tea.
- Brush your teeth.
- Get busy doing something. Before you know it, you'll get to mid-morning, and you can have your snack, plus more broth. Keep in mind your goals, and imagine your body growing lean and healthy during this time.
- Get busy again, and lunch will be here soon! Keep imagining how you want to look, feel, and perform at the end of this short three-week period.
- Get some steady-state exercise during the morning (see more details below). It helps to pass the time, suppress your appetite, and get you better results.

Ultimately, the intermittent fasting is optional, so if you really struggle, then eat a breakfast using ancestral foods (below). There are some breakfast suggestions in the recipe section. You should DEFINITELY skip the morning fast if you are pregnant, breastfeeding, have a history of disordered eating, are very lean, have type I diabetes, and/or struggle with hypoglycemia. You also may need to modify if you exercise at a high intensity in the morning or if you have HPA axis dysfunction (see Who Should Modify—And How on page 74).

Ancestral Foods

Following an ancestral or well-planned paleo diet imparts many health benefits. Some of these include weight loss, improved insulin sensitivity (lower diabetes risk), decreased inflammation (lower risk of heart disease), potent antioxidant and detox support (lower risk of cancer and neurological disease), and improved digestion (helpful for anyone, but especially if you suffer from digestive conditions such as GERD, IBS, IBD, etc).

Ancestral diets are also much lower in the difficult-to-digest proteins that contribute to leaky gut, food sensitivities, and autoimmune disease. There is even a gut-brain connection that is optimized by an ancestral diet. This leads to lower depression and anxiety, as well as improved cognitive function. I could go on, but you get the idea.

Thus, it is essential that you stick to ancestral foods during these twenty-one days. If you get very hungry and need extra food, then please choose items from the following list! These foods will nourish, provide the nutrients your body needs, fight inflammation, and provide healing in many ways.

Ancestral Foods

	Basics	Work Toward	Quality
Protein	Beef, poultry, pork, eggs, fish, and shellfish.	"Nose-to-tail" eating—organ meats, bone broth, bone-in fish (i.e. sardines)—and wild game.	Seek grass-fed meat, wild-caught fish, and free-range poultry/eggs.
Carbohydrates	Starchy vegetables such as sweet and white potatoes, winter squash, parsnips, carrots, taro, and yucca. Also include fresh fruit. Small amounts of natural sweeteners like real, pure maple syrup and raw, local honey.	Never snack on just carbs. Always eat with protein or fat.	Seek organic, especially for fruits with no peel. Look up the EWG's "Clean 15" and "Dirty Dozen" lists for help with prioritizing what produce to purchase organic.
Non-Starchy Vegetables	Any vegetable other than the starchy vegetables listed above. Make this ⅓–½ of your plate, and cook them in ancestral fats when possible.	Increase consumption of fermented vegetables such as sauerkraut, pickles, and kimchi (from the refrigerated section).	Go seasonal and organic when possible. Remember the EWG's "Clean 15" and "Dirty Dozen."
Ancestral Fats and Oils	Coconut oil, coconut milk, grass-fed lard, tallow, or duck fat, extra-virgin olive oil, olives, avocado, avocado oil, ghee, and mayonnaise made with olive or avocado oil.	Incorporate ancestral fats in each meal, and avoid others (see **Avoid** list on the next page).	Get the best quality you can find!

	Basics	Work Toward	Quality
Condiments	Ketchup, mustard, fish sauce, coconut aminos, all-fruit jelly or jam, fish paste, curry paste, salsa, vinegar, oil and vinegar dressing, mayonnaise, horseradish sauce, tartar sauce, real maple syrup, and real honey can all work, depending on the ingredients.	Work on preparing these items at home more often if you can. Preparing your own food gives you the most control in this category. It's nearly impossible to control for this in restaurants.	Try to gradually transition to condiments with fewer additives/preservatives/ingredients. You can even try making your own if you feel ambitious.
Beverages	Lots of water, ideally filtered. Up to 2 cups of black tea or coffee daily. Herbal tea (no limit).	Try to incorporate bone broth and kombucha (fermented tea).	Coffee should be organic and ground at home when possible. Avoid decaffeinated versions of coffee and tea.
Avoid	Absolutely avoid grains of all kinds (wheat, bulgur, couscous, etc.), refined sugar, industrial seed oils (i.e. canola, vegetable, margarine), soy, artificial sweeteners, food additives (i.e. dyes, preservatives, etc.).	Initially eliminate gray area foods; after the challenge, you can slowly try adding them to see how your tolerance fares. These include organic, full-fat dairy (milk, cheese, and yogurt), white rice, stevia, and occasional sprouted legumes (beans).	I know this sounds hard, but it's only twenty-one days. Give it your best shot, and see how you feel; then decide if eating these foods is worth it to you.

Selecting Portion Sizes

If you are following this program for wellness and/or healing, just follow the program and eat the planned foods to satisfy your hunger. However, if you're looking to lose body fat, you will need to be a little more calculated. Start with the below portions, then adjust up or down as needed based on your hunger and weight loss. For meat, I recommend weighing with a food scale. For carbs (fruit or starchy vegetables), make a fist and compare your portion size. Measure fats with a measuring spoon or your thumb. One thumb tip (joint up) = ⅓ Tablespoon (5 ml).

	Lunch/ Dinner Protein	Lunch Carb	Dinner Carb	Fat Serving (all meals)	Snacks: Ancestral Fat & Proteins
Women (low to moderately active)	4 oz (110 g)	½ fist size	½–1 fist size	1 Table-spoon (15 ml)	150–200 calories (see meal plan)
Women (very active) or Men (inac-tive or low activity)	5 oz (140 g)	1 fist size	1 fist size	1–2 Table-spoons (15-30 ml)	200–250 calories (meal plan +50 extra)
Men (very active)	6 oz (170 g)	1 fist size	2 fist size	2+ Table-spoons (30+ ml)	250–300 calories (meal plan +100 extra)

Exercise

I recommend exercise on this plan—and always! Ideally, in the morning you would do some fasted, low-intensity cardio such as walking, swimming, yoga, or cycling. Easy jogging is ok for up to 30 minutes if you are already a runner. Strength training and/or high-intensity exercise should ideally be in the afternoon before your dinner. I know this isn't realistic for everyone, so see modification ideas on page 74.

Dietary Supplements

Recently, a famous functional medicine physician released a new diet book. I was flipping through and all looked good until . . . what?!? You have to buy around $300 of dietary supplements just to follow his twenty-one-day plan! Even worse, some of the supplements recommended could be extremely harmful for some people. Ugh. I *am* very in favor of dietary supplements and use them often in my practice. However, the more you know, the more you realize how careful you have to be. Off-the-shelf brands are often contaminated, don't include what they claim, and/or use the cheap, poorly-absorbed versions of nutrients. Probiotics should be strain-specific for your needs. Vitamin D should be taken as D_3 (cholecalciferol) with vitamin K. The best form of B vitamins for you depends on your methylation status/genetics. Fish oil should be of *high* quality and the right dose, and for many people there are different options that are a better choice. Fermentable fibers can be helpful OR harmful, and more harmful in the case of potato starch. . . . It goes on and on.

So, what does this mean for you? Don't run out and buy a bunch of new supplements. Don't add any new ones. If you have something that works for you, keep it. If you feel like you need help with a "supplement makeover," shoot me an email.

Getting Serious

We're not going for a diet mentality here; we're going for wellness. You might be wondering how strict you need to be. I know life happens. Your family eats the food from your plan, the store doesn't carry something, or you just have a bad day. So, I know 100 percent isn't realistic. However, I recommend getting as close as you can during these twenty-one days. The reason is that this program is designed as a "Reset." I want you loving the way you feel by the end of this. After the twenty-one days you can experiment to find your own personal healthy balance. Some people can be more casual than others depending on many factors: gut health, genetics, medical conditions, lifestyle, age, environment, etc. So, can you give me your all for twenty-one days? After that it's up to you to decide what you can add, starting with the gray area foods from the table on page 71 (see the Avoid row).

Who Should Modify—And How

If you are very active you may struggle with the carbohydrate restriction and fasting of this plan. Ideally, time your workouts as described above. However, let's say you Crossfit or do some other type of high intensity interval training in the *mornings*. I recommend eating around 20–30 g of carbohydrates 30 minutes before your workout, so something like a banana. This pre-workout snack is optional. Some people can exercise fasted better than others. You should have sufficient glycogen storage from your dinner the night prior.

Then, after your workout, eat a snack with 20–30 g carbohydrates and 10 g protein. One example of this is 4 oz (112 g) cooked sweet potato and 2 hard-boiled eggs. Replace your morning snack with this. Adjust your carbohydrate and protein servings at lunch and dinner so that you don't find yourself starving in the evenings. Always eat at least two cups of non-starchy vegetables at each lunch and dinner, ideally with at least ¼ cup fermented vegetables per day. Also, don't forget to have ancestral fat in each meal. Bottom line: if you're starving at night or struggling in the gym, increase the size of your daytime meals and make sure you're fueling properly before and after your workout.

As described above, you should not fast if you are pregnant, breastfeeding, have a history of disordered eating, have type I diabetes, and/or struggle with hypoglycemia. You also may want to skip this if you're already at the right body composition (you don't wish to lose fat). Definitely don't fast if you have a BMI of 19 or below (look online for free calculators). If you train heavily, then I do not recommend fasting on training days. Also, some people just don't feel well doing this. It can be especially problematic if you have HPA axis dysregulation. The common causes are over-stress, under-sleep, over-exercise, and/or chronic illness. If any of those apply to you, ensure that you carefully test your tolerance of intermittent fasting, especially with regard to blood glucose control.

If for any of the above reasons you decide to skip the morning fast, switch to a twelve-hour window. So, if you eat dinner at 6:30 p.m., you can eat breakfast at 6:30 a.m. Just add a breakfast before the morning snack. Use only ancestral foods from the table above, making sure to include fat and/or protein. Some ideas include:

- Scrambled eggs with spinach and avocado
- A smoothie with avocado, fruit, spinach, and coconut milk
- Coconut yogurt with fruit

- A scramble with shredded sweet potato, leftover veggies, eggs, and seasoning
- Egg and veggie "muffins" or "casserole"

I've included a few breakfast recipes in this plan to get you started.

Measuring Progress

Please use at least one of these methods. The important thing is that you record progress in some way consistently.

1. **Weight:** There are some limitations here, but this is the best way for most people. I recommend weighing first thing in the morning, wearing always the same/similar thing or nothing. Please try to wait at least two days between taking weights on this program. Fluctuations are natural but can be discouraging when you see a little upswing. There are apps where you can record your readings, or just write them down. *Record a starting weight the day before you begin.*

2. **Measurements:** This is another great option, especially if you don't like the scale or don't have one. Use a tape measure to record once per week, at the end of each week. Measure with tape taut but not tight and level all around. Get help if you need it. Again, record them in an app or on paper. *Record starting measurements the day before you begin.* Record at least these three locations:
   a. Chest, right at nipple height
   b. Waist, right at your navel
   c. Hips, at the widest point

3. **Clothing Fit:** This is totally fine too. It's pretty gratifying when your old jeans won't stay up. Please keep a written or typed diary, and make an entry of how you feel/look weekly (before you start, then at the end of each week).

4. **Lab Markers:** If you are looking to improve a physiological marker such as your lipid panel or glucose control, then make sure to get baseline labs before you begin.

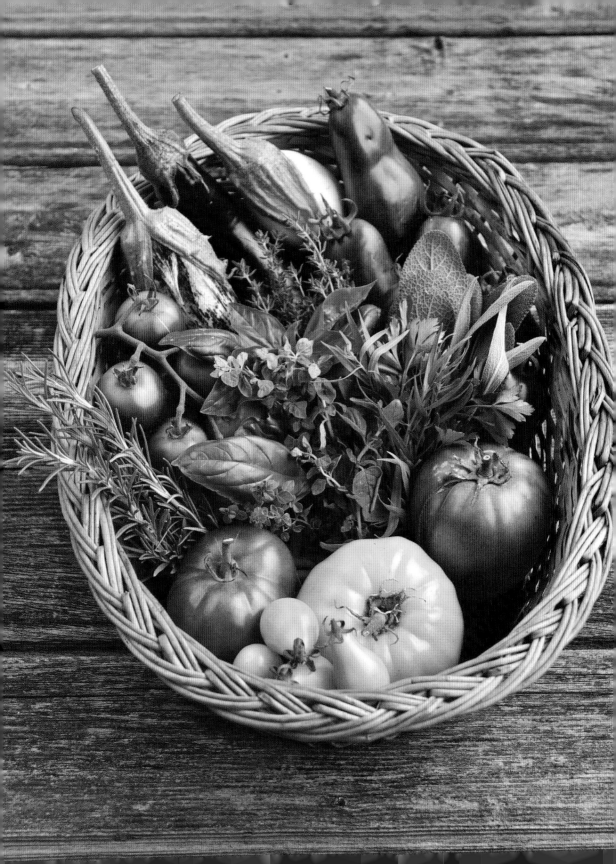

10

Meal Plans
and
Shopping Lists

It's your choice if you'd like to follow the meal plans, design your own meals, or do a combination of the two. I find that people usually have better success if they follow the meal plans. If you (or your family) are not big on leftovers, just add some additional recipes to your plan for the week. Check the Resources section on page 192 for some great recipe sources.

Week 1: Meal Plan

NO: Grains, dairy, legumes, soy, refined sugar, refined fats/industrial seed oils

	Day 1	Day 2	Day 3
Breakfast	1 cup hot, salted broth	1 cup hot, salted broth	1 cup hot, salted broth
A.M. Snack	2 hard-boiled eggs (or cook how you like) + 1 cup hot, salted broth	¼ cup (2 oz/56 g) raw sunflower seeds + 1 cup hot, salted broth	2 hard-boiled eggs (or cook how you like) + 1 cup hot, salted broth
Lunch	Curried Tuna Salad (eat half recipe—save leftovers—on 2 cups mixed greens, 1 chopped tomato, ½ cucumber, sliced) + 1 cup fresh berries	Leftovers: 4–6oz chicken from Whole Chicken Broth w/S&P + 2 cups steamed, salted broccoli florets + 1 peach or nectarine	Leftovers: Curried Tuna Salad (on 2 cups mixed greens, 1 chopped tomato, ½ cucumber, sliced) + 1 cup fresh berries
P.M. Snack	¼ cup (2 oz/56 g) raw or dry-roasted cashews	¼ cup (2 oz/56 g) unsweetened coconut chips/flakes	¼ cup (2 oz/56 g) raw or dry-roasted cashews
Dinner	4–6oz chicken from Whole Chicken Broth w/S&P + 2 cups steamed, salted broccoli florets + 3–5 oz cooked sweet potato with 1 tsp ghee	1–2 servings Bone Broth Chicken Curry + ⅓ recipe Super Quick Cauilfower Rice + ½ mango	Leftovers: 1–2 servings Bone Broth Chicken Curry + ⅓ recipe Super Quick Cauilfower Rice + ½ mango. *Start Legit Beef Bone Broth* (will be ready tomorrow).*

Recipes: Whole Chicken Broth, Curried Tuna Salad, Bone Broth Chicken Curry, Super Quick Cauliflower Rice, Low-Carb Braised Beef, Supercharged Mashed Veg, Legit Beef Bone Broth, Super Food Soup
NOTE: May have up to 2 cups coffee or tea per day. May add 1 Tbsp almond milk and a little stevia if desired. Unlimited herbal tea OK. Try to add ¼ cup fermented veggies each day.

Day 4	Day 5	Day 6	Day 7
1 cup hot, salted broth	1 cup hot, salted broth	1 cup hot, salted broth	1 cup hot, salted broth
¼ cup (2 oz/56 g) raw sunflower seeds + 1 cup hot, salted broth	2 hard-boiled eggs (or cook how you like) + 1 cup hot, salted broth	¼ cup (2 oz/56 g) raw sunflower seeds + 1 cup hot, salted broth	2 hard-boiled eggs (or cook how you like) + 1 cup hot, salted broth
Leftovers: 1–2 servings Bone Broth Chicken Curry + ⅓ recipe Super Quick Cauliflower Rice + 1 peach or nectarine (freeze any remaining leftover curry)	Leftovers: Super Food Soup + salad (2 cups baby spinach, 1 chopped tomato, ⅓ bell pepper, thinly sliced red onion, ⅓ cucumber, sliced, and 1 Tbsp oil & vinegar dressing)	Leftovers: Super Food Soup + salad (2 cups baby spinach, 1 chopped tomato, ⅓ bell pepper, thinly sliced red onion, ⅓ cucumber, sliced, and 1 Tbsp oil & vinegar dressing)	Leftovers: 4–6 oz Low-Carb Braised Beef with 1–2 cups veggies from recipe + ½–1 cup Supercharged Mashed Veg (freeze leftovers)
¼ cup (2 oz/56 g) unsweetened coconut chips/flakes	¼ cup (2 oz/56 g) raw or dry-roasted cashews	¼ cup (2 oz/56 g) unsweetened coconut chips/flakes	¼ cup (2 oz/56 g) raw or dry-roasted cashews
Super Food Soup + salad (2 cups baby spinach, 1 chopped tomato, ⅓ bell pepper, thinly sliced red onion, ⅓ cucumber, sliced, and 1 Tbsp oil & vinegar dressing)	**START EARLY: 4–6 oz Low-Carb Braised Beef with 1–2 cups veggies from recipe + ½–1 cup Supercharged Mashed Veg	Leftovers: 4–6 oz Low-Carb Braised Beef with 1–2 cups veggies from recipe + ½–1 cup Supercharged Mashed Veg	Enjoy a clean meal out, finish leftovers from the week, or make a simple dinner of your choice.

*If you make Legit Beef Bone Broth with a slow cooker, you may not have enough to finish out the week. Either make in a large stock pot (with at least 4 quarts/liters of water), or save bones to use in a second batch.

**Day 5 dinner (Low-Carb Braised Beef) needs to braise ~4 hours. Plan ahead for this, *or* may swap with soup if needed.

Week 1: Grocery List

Meat, Poultry & Eggs	
8	Eggs
1	Whole organic chicken (large if possible; must fit in your crock pot with lid closed)
2 lb (1 kg)	Boneless, skinless chicken thighs
4–6 lbs (2–3 kg)	Grass-fed beef bones (if possible: half marrow and/or knuckle bones and half meaty such as short ribs and/or shanks)
~4 lbs (2 kg)	Beef chuck roast, pot roast, roasting joint, or other large, tough beef roast (may go half-size if needed for cost)
NOTE: Buy grass-fed, free-range, and organic whenever possible.	

Produce	
2 cups	Fresh berries of choice (blueberries, strawberries, raspberries, etc.)
2	Peaches or nectarines
1	Medium ripe mango
2	Green apples
4 cups	Mixed salad greens
6 cups	Baby spinach (for salad)
1	Bell pepper (any color, for salad)
5	Medium vine-ripe tomatoes
2	Cucumbers
8	Carrots
1 lb (450 g)	Parsnips (may substitute other root vegetable)
2	Celery bunches
3	Zucchini (aka: courgette)
1 large head	Broccoli

(continued)

Produce	
1 head	Cauliflower (or 2 if they're small)
½ head	Green or white cabbage
1	Butternut squash (may use ~2 lb/1 kg pre-peeled, chopped cubes)
4 cups	Mushrooms
2	Medium sweet potatoes (3–5 oz each)
2 lb (1 kg)	White potatoes (may substitute sweet potatoes)
6	Baby white potatoes (may substitute ~2 sweet potatoes)
1	Red onion
8	Medium white or yellow onions
2–3 bulbs	Garlic (20 cloves)
6 sprigs	Fresh thyme (1 bunch)
4 sprigs	Fresh parsley (1 bunch)
2 sprigs	Fresh rosemary (may substitute dried)
1 piece	Fresh ginger (will need 3 Tablespoons chopped)
NOTE: Buy organic, especially for items without peel, whenever possible.	

"Dairy"	
1 carton	Nut or coconut milk (if needed for tea/coffee)
NOTE: Buy organic if at all possible. Avoid carrageenan in nut milks.	

Canned Goods	
1 can	Coconut milk (full fat)
1 6-oz can (56 g)	Tuna (packed in water)
1 28-oz can (840 ml)	Chopped tomatoes

Spices & Condiments	
3 Tbsp	Ghee (clarified butter)
3 Tbsp	Olive oil and vinegar dressing (clean ingredients or make own)
1 Tbsp	Balsamic vinegar
½ cup	Apple cider vinegar (aka: cider vinegar, ACV)
2 Tbsp	Avocado oil- or olive oil-mayonnaise
5 Tbsp	Coconut oil
1 Tbsp	Duck fat (or substitute more coconut oil)
2 tsp	Fish sauce (clean ingredients)
½ tsp	Ground coriander
½ tsp	Ground cumin
1 tsp	Ground nutmeg
1 tsp	Ground turmeric
1½ Tbsp	Curry powder
4	Bay leaves
	Sea salt and black pepper
	Stevia for tea/coffee (optional)
NOTE: Change up the use of spices in the recipes according to your liking. If you don't have a lot of the spices listed, feel free to omit some or substitute to keep costs down.	

Beverages	
Drink only water and up to two cups of coffee and/or tea per day. Unlimited herbal tea OK.	
8–10 qts (2½ gal)	Filtered water (bottled or home-filtered)
2 cups (480 ml)	Red wine (optional) (for Low-Carb Braised Beef recipe on page 175)

Snacks	
¾ cup (3 oz/90 g)	Raw sunflower seeds
1 cup (4 oz/112 g)	Raw or dry-roasted cashews
3 Tbsp	Crushed walnuts (optional garnish)
4 oz (112 g)	Unsweetened coconut chips or flakes (check bulk bins, health food stores, online)
2 cups	Fermented veggies from refrigerated section, such as sauerkraut, kimchi, pickles, etc. (optional) (Try to include ¼ cup fermented veggies every day.)

Abbreviations & Conversions
Tbsp = Tablespoon = 15 ml
tsp = teaspoon = 5 ml
cup = 8 oz = 240 ml (liquid)

Prep for Day 1

1. Make Whole Chicken Broth the day before you begin. You'll need it for the first morning of Week 1!
2. Hard-boil 8 eggs (place eggs in pot filled with cold water, bring to boil, turn off heat, leave covered 12 minutes, drain, and cool in cold water).
3. Plan ahead. You'll need a source for your beef bones and organic chicken (for broth).

Week 2: Meal Plan

NO: Grains, dairy, legumes, soy, refined sugar, refined fats/industrial seed oils

	Day 1	Day 2	Day 3
Breakfast	1 cup hot, salted broth	1 cup hot, salted broth	1 cup hot, salted broth
A.M. Snack	¼ cup (2 oz/56 g) raw or dry-roasted macadamia nuts + 1 cup hot, salted broth	⅕ recipe #SoGood Chia Pudding + 1 cup hot, salted broth	¼ cup (2 oz/56 g) raw or dry-roasted macadamia nuts + 1 cup hot, salted broth
Lunch	Antipasto lunch: 1 oz salami slices, 1 oz prosciutto, 10 green olives, salad (1 chopped tomato, ½ cucumber, sliced, S&P, and 1 Tbsp oil & vinegar dressing) + 1 cup berries	Leftover Quickie Roast Chicken (4–6 oz chicken + 1–1½ cups carrot/parsnip)	Leftover Quickie Roast Chicken (4–6 oz chicken + 1–1½ cups carrot/parsnip)
P.M. Snack	Avocado To Go	¼ cup (2 oz/56 g) clean beef or turkey jerky	Avocado To Go
Dinner	Quickie Roast Chicken (DOUBLE recipe): eat 4–6 oz chicken + 1–1½ cups carrot/parsnip. *Remove/save all meat and start Inflammation-Fighting Broth (needed for Day 4; make this on Day 2 or 3 if you have enough other broth for breakfast/snacks).*	Breakfast for dinner! Eat 1 serving Banana Pancakes, topped with 1 Tbsp almond butter. May eat 1–2 extra eggs, cooked separately, if high-activity level. *Make A Little Something Broth (needed for tomorrow).*	1–2 servings Re-Mix Chili over 1 cup Roasted Squash Noodles

Recipes: Quickie Roast Chicken, Inflammation-Fighting Broth, Supercharged Greens, Healing Chicken Soup, Banana Pancakes, A Little Something Broth, Re-Mix Chili, Roasted Squash Noodles, Sunny Day Fish, Avocado To Go, #SoGood Chia Pudding

Day 4	Day 5	Day 6	Day 7
1 cup hot, salted broth	1 cup hot, salted broth	1 cup hot, salted broth	1 cup hot, salted broth
⅓ recipe #SoGood Chia Pudding + 1 cup hot, salted broth	¼ cup (2 oz/56 g) raw or dry-roasted macadamia nuts + 1 cup hot, salted broth	⅓ recipe #So-Good Chia Pudding + 1 cup hot, salted broth	¼ cup (2 oz/56 g) raw or dry-roasted macadamia nuts + 1 cup hot, salted broth
Leftovers: 1–2 servings Re-Mix Chili over 1 cup Roasted Squash Noodles	Leftovers: 1–2 servings Re-Mix Chili over 1 cup Roasted Squash Noodles	Leftovers: 1 serving Healing Chicken Soup + 1 serving Supercharged Greens + 1 plum	Antipasto lunch: 1 oz salami slices, 1 oz prosciutto, 10 green olives, salad (1 chopped tomato, ½ cucumber, sliced, S&P, and 1 Tbsp oil & vinegar dressing) + 1 cup berries
¼ cup (2 oz/56 g) clean beef or turkey jerky	Avocado To Go	¼ cup (2 oz/56 g) clean beef or turkey jerky	Avocado To Go
1 serving Healing Chicken Soup (use Inflammation-Fighting Broth and all leftover chicken, may add more from rotisserie chicken if needed) + 1 serving Supercharged Greens + 1 plum	Leftovers: 1 serving Healing Chicken Soup + 1 serving Supercharged Greens + 1 plum	1 serving Sunny Day Fish + 10–20 spears steamed, salted asparagus + 3–5 oz baked sweet potato with 1 tsp ghee	Leftovers: 1 serving Sunny Day Fish + 10–20 spears steamed, salted asparagus + 3–5 oz baked sweet potato with 1 tsp ghee

NOTE: May have up to 2 cups coffee or tea per day. May add 1 Tbsp almond milk and a little stevia if desired. Unlimited herbal tea OK. Try to add ¼ cup fermented veggies each day.

Week 2: Grocery List

	Meat, Poultry, Seafood & Eggs
6	Eggs
1	Rotisserie chicken
2	Roasting chickens (~3–5 lbs/1½ –2½ kg each; may go smaller or even just buy one if feeding only 1–2 people)
1 lb (450 g)	Grass-fed beef
4–6 lbs (2–3 kg)	Beef bones (if possible: half marrow and/or knuckle bones and half meaty such as short ribs and/or shanks)
1 lb (450 g)	Sea bass fillets (or tilapia, halibut, pollock, mahi mahi, cod, or sole)
6 slices	American "streaky" bacon
2 oz (60 g)	Salami slices (check ingredients for quality)
2 oz (60 g)	Prosciutto (may substitute other clean, cured meat if needed)
NOTE: Buy grass-fed, free-range, and organic whenever possible. For seafood, look for wild-caught.	

	Produce
2 cups	Fresh berries of choice
3	Plums
2	Ripe bananas
2	Avocados
1	Medium orange
2	Lemons
1 large bunch	Winter greens (collard, chard, kale, etc.)
2	Bell peppers (any color)
1	Jalapeño pepper (optional)
1 lb (450 g)	Asparagus spears

(continued)

Produce	
2 cups	Sliced mushrooms
6	Medium vine-ripe tomatoes
1	Cucumber
1 head	Celery
21	Medium carrots
8	Parsnips (may substitute other root vegetable as needed)
2	Medium sweet potatoes (6–10 oz/170–300 g total)
8	Medium white or yellow onions
4 heads	Garlic (need 2 whole, unbroken heads + 16 cloves)
1	Spaghetti squash (may substitute other winter squash as needed)
1 bunch	Green onions (or scallions or chives) (optional garnish)
1 bunch	Fresh dill (may substitute dried)
1 bunch	Fresh parsley
3 bunches	Fresh thyme (or buy 1 large bunch and split)
NOTE: Buy organic, especially for items without peel, whenever possible.	

"Dairy"	
1 carton	Nut or coconut milk (if needed for tea/coffee)
NOTE: Buy organic if at all possible. Avoid carrageenan in nut milks.	

Canned Goods	
1 can	Coconut milk (full fat)
1 14-oz can (~400 g)	Crushed tomatoes
1 14-oz can (~400 g)	Diced tomatoes
1 4-oz can (~120 g)	Diced green chiles (may substitute other fresh/jarred/canned hot chili) (optional)

Spices & Condiments	
7 Tbsp	Ghee
5 Tbsp	Coconut oil
3 Tbsp	Olive oil
½ cup	Apple cider vinegar
2 Tbsp	Olive oil & vinegar dressing (can make at home, or buy a clean-ingredients version)
1 Tbsp	Dijon mustard
3 Tbsp	Honey, raw, local if possible
1 Tbsp	Almond butter (or other nut-/seed butter—*not* peanut)
3	whole allspice berries (may substitute ½ tsp ground allspice), *or* ½ tsp ground cinnamon + ⅛ tsp ground cloves (may substitute 3 whole cloves)
4	Bay leaves
¼ tsp	Ground cardamom (optional)
⅛ tsp	Cayenne pepper (optional)
1 Tbsp	Chili powder
2 tsp	Cinnamon
2 tsp	Ground cumin
2 tsp	Garlic powder (check ingredients; avoid fillers)
1 tsp	Paprika
2 tsp	Ground turmeric
	Sea salt and black pepper
¼ cup	Chia seeds (whole, *not* milled)
2 tsp	Real vanilla extract
⅛ tsp	Baking powder
	Stevia for tea/coffee (optional)
NOTE: Change up the use of spices in the recipes according to your liking. If you don't have a lot of the spices listed, feel free to omit some or substitute to keep costs down.	

Beverages	
Drink only water and up to two cups of coffee and/or tea per day. Unlimited herbal tea OK.	
8–10 qts (2½ gal)	Filtered water (bottled or home-filtered)

Snacks	
1 cup (4 oz/112 g)	Raw or dry-roasted macadamia nuts (may substitute other tree nuts)
6 oz (170 g)	Clean beef jerky (may use turkey)
20	Green olives (may substitute black olives) (can be from deli counter or canned)
2 cups	Fermented veggies from refrigerated section, such as sauerkraut, kimchi, pickles, etc. (optional) (Try to include ¼ cup fermented veggies every day.)
½ cup	Coconut butter (aka: coconut manna, coconut cream concentrate, or creamed coconut—*not* coconut oil) (You'll actually need this for Week 3, but you might need to order ahead online. Alternately, you may skip this and substitute a snack from previous weeks.)

Abbreviations & Conversions
Tbsp = Tablespoon = 15 ml
tsp = teaspoon = 5 ml
cup = 8 oz = 240 ml (liquid)

Prep for Day 1

1. You may want to purchase kitchen string for roasting chickens if you don't already have it at home.

Week 3: Meal Plan

NO: Grains, dairy, legumes, soy, refined sugar, refined fats/industrial seed oils

	Day 1	Day 2	Day 3
Break-fast	1 cup hot, salted broth	1 cup hot, salted broth	1 cup hot, salted broth
A.M. Snack	¼ cup (2 oz/56 g/15-count) almonds (no oil) + 1 cup hot, salted broth	1 scrambled or hard-boiled egg with 2 oz (56 g) lox + 1 cup hot, salted broth	¼ cup (2 oz/56 g/15-count) almonds (no oil) + 1 cup hot, salted broth
Lunch	"Brunch": Stir-fry 1 cup spinach and 1 diced to-mato, scramble 2 eggs in this, serve topped with ½ avocado, sliced + 1 small or ½ medi-um-large grapefruit on side	Leftovers: 4–6oz beef + 2 cups steamed, salted broccoli + 1 serving Addicting Sweet Potato Fries	Leftovers: 4–6oz beef + 2 cups steamed, salted broccoli + 1 serving Addicting Sweet Potato Fries
P.M. Snack	3 Chocolate Coconut Balls (¼ recipe)	¼ cup (2 oz/56 g) pumpkin seeds	3 Chocolate Coconut Balls (¼ recipe)
Dinner	Make Drink Your Broth and Eat It Too (start early!). Eat 4–6oz beef + 2 cups steamed, salt-ed broccoli + 1 serving Addicting Sweet Potato Fries	1 serving Sweet & Spicy Wings + 2 ju-lienned raw carrots + 3 celery stalks (cut in thirds) + 2 Tbsp Cleaned-Up Ranch. *Save bones!*	1 serving Maple Roast Salmon + 1 serving Bacon-Roasted Sprouts + 1 medium orange

Recipes: Drink Your Broth and Eat It Too, Addicting Sweet Potato Fries, Sweet & Spicy Wings, Cleaned-Up Ranch, Bacon-Roasted Sprouts, Good Fats Chicken Salad, Baba Ganoush Lamb with Zucchini Noodles, Chocolate Coconut Balls, Chopped Pesto Salad, Maple Roast Salmon, Whole Chicken Broth

Day 4	Day 5	Day 6	Day 7
1 cup hot, salted broth	1 cup hot, salted broth	1 cup hot, salted broth	1 cup hot, salted broth
1 scrambled or hard-boiled egg with 2 oz (56 g) lox + 1 cup hot, salted broth	¼ cup (2 oz/56 g/ 15-count) almonds (no oil) + 1 cup hot, salted broth	1 scrambled or hard-boiled egg with 2 oz (56 g) lox + 1 cup hot, salted broth	¼ cup (2 oz/56 g/ 15-count) almonds (no oil) + 1 cup hot, salted broth
Leftovers: 1 serving Sweet & Spicy Wings + 2 julienned raw carrots + 3 celery stalks (cut in thirds) + 2 Tbsp Cleaned-Up Ranch. *Save bones!*	Leftovers: 1 serving Maple Roast Salmon + 1 serving Bacon-Roasted Sprouts + 1 medium orange	1 serving Chopped Pesto Salad (use leftover chicken) on 2 cups salad greens + 1 small pear	1 serving Chopped Pesto Salad (use leftover chicken) on 2 cups salad greens + 1 small pear
¼ cup (2 oz/56 g) pumpkin seeds	3 Chocolate Coconut Balls (¼ recipe)	¼ cup (2 oz/56 g) pumpkin seeds	3 Chocolate Coconut Balls (¼ recipe)
Leftovers: 1 serving Maple Roast Salmon + 1 serving Bacon-Roasted Sprouts + 1 medium orange	Make Whole Chicken Broth using whole chicken and leftover wing bones (start in a.m.). Use chicken to make Good Fats Chicken Salad (eat 1 recipe/ serving). Make pesto for tomorrow if necessary.	1 serving (⅓ recipe) Baba Ganoush Lamb with Zucchini Noodles. 1 small square dark chocolate *(Finish line—you earned it!)*	1 serving (⅓ recipe) Baba Ganoush Lamb with Zucchini Noodles. 1 small square dark chocolate *(Finish line—you earned it!)*

NOTE: May have up to 2 cups coffee or tea each day. May add 1 Tbsp almond milk and a little stevia if desired. Unlimited herbal tea OK. Try to add ¼ cup fermented veggies each day. Lox = smoked salmon.

Week 3: Grocery List

Meat, Poultry, Seafood & Eggs	
5	Eggs
1	Whole chicken (3–4 lbs/1½–2 kg)
2 lb (1 kg)	Bone-in chicken wings
4–6 lbs (2–3 kg)	Beef shanks, or 2–4 lb (1–2 kg) tough beef roast + ~4lb (2 kg) beef bones
1 lb (450 g)	Ground lamb (may substitute ground beef)
6 oz (170 g)	Lox (smoked salmon)
1 lb (450 g)	Fresh salmon
6 pieces	American "streaky" bacon
NOTE: Buy grass-fed, free-range, and organic whenever possible. For seafood, look for wild-caught.	

Produce	
1	Medium apple
2	Small pears
1	Small grapefruit (or ½ medium-large grapefruit)
3	Medium oranges
1	Lime
1	Avocado
1 cup	Spinach leaves, fresh
7 cups	Mixed salad greens (your choice) (may want to buy late in the week, when they're actually called for)
3	Medium vine-ripe tomatoes
10	Large carrots
2 heads	Celery (need 11 stalks)
1½ lb (700 g)	Brussels sprouts

(continued)

Produce	
2 large heads	Broccoli
2	Medium eggplants (aka: aubergine) (or 1 large)
2	Medium zucchini (aka: courgette)
1 lb (450 g)	Sweet potatoes
4	Medium white or yellow onions
1 head	Garlic (need 11 cloves)
2	Green onions (or scallions or spring onions)
4 cups	Fresh basil leaves
2 sprigs	Fresh dill
3 Tbsp	Fresh mint
2 sprigs	Fresh parsley
2 sprigs	Fresh rosemary
4 sprigs	Fresh thyme
1 piece	Ginger root (~1 inch)
NOTE: Buy organic, especially for items without peel, whenever possible.	

"Dairy"	
1 carton	Nut or coconut milk (if needed for tea/coffee)
NOTE: Buy organic if at all possible. Avoid carrageenan in nut milks.	

Canned Goods	
1 can	Coconut milk (full fat)
1 14-oz can (~400 g)	Crushed tomatoes (may substitute chopped tomatoes)
1 jar	Roasted red peppers (will actually only need 2 large pieces of the red pepper)
1 jar	Green chilies (will actually only need 2 of the green chilies) (may substitute 1 jalapeño) (optional)

Spices & Condiments	
½ cup	Olive oil
½ tsp	White vinegar
1¼ cups	Apple cider vinegar
½ cup	Avocado oil (may substitute olive oil-mayonnaise)
5 Tbsp	Coconut oil
2 Tbsp + 1 tsp	Coconut aminos (may substitute fish sauce) (optional)
2 Tbsp	Honey, raw, local if possible
¾ cup	Pure maple syrup
2 Tbsp	Dijon mustard
1 jar	Chermoula paste (will actually only need 4 Tbsp) (may make your own with recipe on page 187)
4	Bay leaves
1 stick	Cinnamon (or ¼ tsp ground)
¼ tsp	Ground cloves
½ tsp	Onion powder
½ tsp	Dried oregano
½ tsp	Paprika
1 tsp	Pumpkin pie spice (may substitute cinnamon) (optional)
½ tsp	Red pepper flakes (may substitute cayenne) (optional)
1 tsp	Ground turmeric (or use fresh root)
	Sea salt and black pepper
1 tsp	Real vanilla extract
1 Tbsp	Cocoa powder
	Stevia for tea/coffee (optional)
NOTE: Change up the use of spices in the recipes according to your liking. If you don't have a lot of the spices listed, feel free to omit some or substitute to keep costs down.	

Beverages	
Drink only water and up to two cups of coffee and/or tea per day. Unlimited herbal tea OK.	
8–10 qts (2½ gal)	Filtered water (bottled or home-filtered)

Snacks	
2 small squares	Dark chocolate
4 oz (120 g)	Almonds (*not* roasted in oil)
2 Tbsp	Crushed walnuts
½ cup	Raw pine nuts
¾ cup (90 g)	Raw or dry roasted pumpkin seeds
½ cup	Unsweetened, shredded coconut (or flakes)
½ cup	Coconut butter (aka: coconut manna, coconut cream concentrate, or creamed coconut—*not* coconut oil) (You may have already bought/ordered this during Week 2. Alternately, you may skip this and substitute a snack from previous weeks.)
2 cups	Fermented veggies from refrigerated section, such as sauerkraut, kimchi, pickles, etc. (optional) (Try to include ¼ cup fermented veggies every day.)

Abbreviations & Conversions
Tbsp = Tablespoon = 15 ml
tsp = teaspoon = 5 ml
cup = 8 oz = 240 ml (liquid)

Meal Plan FAQ

You can use the meal plans for the program, *or* use the template from Chapter 9 to plan your own meals. However, I find that people usually have the best success with meal plans. They are *especially* helpful in this program because I've lined you up to make batches of broth, then use that broth in your dinner recipes! That way you're getting the ideal 2–3 cups per day. Also, it's just nice to have it all planned out and not have to think about it. Pretend you have your own personal dietitian for three weeks. Enjoy it!

Here are some common questions when it comes to following the meal plans:

1. How do I know how much bone broth to make?
If you use a slow cooker to make your broth, you might not have enough for the meal plan—*especially* with beef broth. This problem is even possible with stock pots. It depends on the size of your slow cooker or pot and of the bones (beef bones displace more water). I recommend that (especially the first week) you quick-turn your beef bones. So, make the broth recipe, save the bones, then put them right back in for a second batch. You can use less or even *no* veg/herbs/spices if you need to. The vinegar is mandatory. Once you have a "broth stash," you can relax and stop making double-batches.

2. Can I make some meals early in the week and refrigerate or freeze for later?
Yes, that's no problem! Bone broth also freezes beautifully, so feel free to make up a bunch right at the beginning if you have the space.

3. I didn't like a meal and it repeats later in the week! What should I do?
Feel free to substitute another meal from the plan of the same type (i.e. snacks can replace snacks, lunches can replace lunches, etc). Also, feel free to change spices/seasonings as you wish for all menu items. The same goes for garnishes such as capers.

4. What if I don't like a food (i.e. fish) from the plan?
You can substitute proteins however you like, as long as you use the same amounts. So, if the meal plan says to eat 4 ounces of fish, eat 4 ounces of something like chicken breast instead. If there is a different type of fish or seafood (i.e. shellfish) you like, that's even better (there are important nutrients obtained almost exclusively from seafood). Substitute starchy carbs for similar vegetables—

and the same goes for fruits, non-starchy vegetables, and fats (see the Ancestral Foods table on page 70 for help with which foods belong to each group).

5. Can I eat the meals out of order?
Yes, it's not a problem to change around which days you eat which meals. Please do try to follow the meal order though. In other words, still follow the pattern of broth, broth/snack, lunch, snack, dinner each day. Try not to skip meals then eat them all at once later, and try not to skip them altogether. Remember to shoot for that 15–18-hour fasting window between dinner and a.m. snack (or lunch if you skip a.m. snack).

6. Why can't I skip snacks or meals?
We're shooting for the sweet spot between getting the benefits of intermittent fasting and getting enough nutrition during our eating window. Since you're having a fasting window every day, you don't want to make it too long. Rather than skipping snacks or meals, look to adjust your serving sizes using the "Selecting Portion Sizes" table (on page 72) as a starting place. Let me know if you need help. [Insert a new paragraph]

7. How big should my serving be?
I don't recommend weighing the final serving of a recipe because the weight will vary depending on many factors—including the size of the produce (e.g., how big your cauliflower head was), how much water your produce naturally contained, how much liquid was cooked off, and so on. Instead, I find that my clients get better control by carefully weighing and measuring the protein and fat ingredients of the recipe during the preparation stage and then eating a fraction of the final yield. So, for example, you may make a salmon meal with the correct weight of salmon and the correct amount of fat according to the recipe. Then, look to the meal plan to determine how much to eat (e.g., the plan may say to eat 1 serving of 4, or ¼ of the yield). Another benefit of this approach is that you will have the correct number of servings to match the meal plan—not too many leftovers and not too few. This prevents food waste and keeps you from scrambling to find a substitute.

8. What if I'm cooking for more than just myself?
This is important. The amounts listed on the grocery list are only for one person. If you will be preparing meals for additional people, make sure to buy extra groceries! For example, my husband eats breakfast and lunch at work so I keep those as planned. However, our whole family eats dinner together. So, before I shop, I look

at what proteins and veggies are on the dinners for the week. I buy at least double of those, plus extra for other meals I will make (e.g., breakfast for my children). It's better to make too much than too little, so that you have an easy day with leftovers when the plan calls for it. If you end up with uneaten servings, you can freeze those for after the plan.

9. Help—I'm trying to scale up these recipes for additional people, but now it's hard to figure out how much to eat!
Again, if you are not pursuing a weight loss goal, you can just eat to satisfy your hunger. If you want to be more calculated, then use the "Selecting Portion Sizes" table (on page 72) to help you figure out how much of your yield to eat. Here is the basic technique I recommend:

- Figure out how much would be a protein serving. So, if you used 2 pounds (32 oz) meat, and you need a 4 oz serving, then you should eat ⅛ of your yield.
- Look at the table and see if it includes 2+ cups of non-starchy vegetables (i.e., a stir-fry might). If not, add these.
- Look at the table again to see what carb serving you need. If you don't already have this on your plate (riding with the meat entrée), add it. Fruit works well in a pinch, or use non-starchy vegetables.
- Got some fat already riding in any of those? Good to go. If not, add some. Olive oil, ghee, coconut milk, or nut butters are the easiest to add.

A Note on Units
If you are using the meal plans and shopping lists, I have tried to provide both US and metric units where possible. However, if you don't usually use US measurements (i.e. cups and teaspoons), you can consult the list below as well as the chart at the back of this book. Most food scales allow you to change units between grams and ounces, so that can be helpful at home. It's also helpful to use an app or website to convert units easily. Here are some basic conversions that I find helpful:

1 lb = 450 g
1 oz = 28 g
2.2 lbs = 1 kg
1 Tablespoon (Tbsp) = 15 ml
1 teaspoon (tsp) = 5 ml
1 cup = 8 fluid oz = 240 ml

11

Success on the Bone Both Miracle Diet

I've helped hundreds of people change their lives by implementing an ancestral diet. If there's one thing I've learned, it's that just knowing the facts isn't enough. If you want to get great results from this program, you'll need the mind-set to go with it. In this chapter, I'd like to go over four concepts that are *key* to having a mind-set for success.

1. Your Personal Motivation

The first is motivation. Eating clean for twenty-one days is a lot harder than it sounds. To be consistent, you'll need to know the answer to one question: "What is your motivator?"

Because here's the thing: we all start out with good intentions. But then life happens. A "slip-up." We get derailed. How we react to these moments is critical, and our reaction has everything to do with *what* motivates us. I find that not only do we need to know what it is, but we need to know *specifics*.

Keeping our specific goals in mind is what keeps us from giving in to a craving, giving up, or only giving half our effort.

So, what is it for you?

- Are you looking to improve lab values? *What* value, and to what level? What medical condition are you looking to avoid or improve? For what reason? Longevity, quality of life, family?
- Do you want to lose body fat? Why, and what will it look/feel like? What will people say, and how will they react? How will your clothes fit? How will your health improve?

- Are you trying to improve symptoms? How so? What will it feel like to live without the aches, pains, bloating, gas, allergies, migraines, brain fog . . . what is it for you? What new things will you be able to do without those symptoms?

You get the idea. We need to get down to the *root* of our motivation and to keep that thing at the *forefront* of our mind. In fact, I recommend journaling on this topic at least three times per week during the program. Write down your thoughts, what you want to achieve, and renew your commitment.

Although it might sound like it, this is *not* meant to be a message that you just need to "diet harder." I'm very anti-diet, in fact. The truth is that I want to help you find true wellness, an eating style that makes you thrive, and to make it EASY.

I find that only when people experience the absolute physical REVOLUTION of eating a well-planned ancestral diet do they realize its power. For that reason, I encourage you to commit 100 percent for these twenty-one days. Then, see how you feel, and go from there. Figure out your own best balance.

2. The Diet Mentality

Speaking of anti-dieting . . . I learned a pretty insane statistic the other day. Guess how many diets the average woman has been on by the age of 45. Sixty-one. SIXTY-ONE diets. That's around two per year from the age of sixteen on.

Are you surprised?

Maybe not very, actually. Diet culture is everywhere. Despite this, rates of overweight and obesity continue to rise. Most diets only last fifteen days on average, and 35 percent of dieters *gain* weight during the course of the diet! Hmmm, I wonder why. I opened a really popular magazine the other day and saw (of course) a weight loss diet. The recommendations? Diet soda. Fast-food chain salad. 100-calorie cookie bags. Are you *kidding* me? What a recipe for disaster.

So, I hope you believe me when I say that I am anti-diet. I am pro-wellness. I truly believe that the reason why people try to diet so often is that their baseline diet is poor. No amount of dieting can make up for *not knowing the right way to eat*.

And it's not your fault. The standard nutrition message is so confused and, frankly, wrong. There are government guidelines encouraging grains, industrial oils, soy, and fat-free dairy. There are diet evangelists swearing that their extreme version of detox, vegan, no-carb, bio-hacking coffee, macro counting, whatever . . . is the only answer. To be honest, even the professionals are confused. If you aren't confused as well, you're probably just not paying close attention (that's probably wise of you).

I know that I'm asking you to be very strict for these twenty-one days. That is because I want you to feel and see the results that you can get from eating well. Once you've experienced that and have learned to do it with ease, life can go on—feeling and looking great—*without diets*. So please don't feel like I'm trying to tell you to "diet harder." I'm genuinely trying to help you reset . . . on the way to a healthy life of *non-dieting*.

3. Non-Dieting vs. Cravings

This brings us to a bit of a difficult place. We want to ditch our old dieting mentality, but we *do* want to experience a twenty-one-day wellness revolution. So, how do we address it when we get a craving for something that's not a part of the program?

By a large margin, the most common cravings are for sweets. It feels like lately every client I have reports major cravings for sweets. The traditional advice? Eat them in moderation. I find that sometimes that helps and sometimes it doesn't. Often, the more sugar we eat, the more we want. So, going cold turkey for a period of time can really help—that's the goal with this program.

Really, cravings can have quite a variety of causes. Here are a few:

- Lack of sleep
- Under-hydration
- Stress—emotional or physical (e.g., over-exercise or chronic disease)
- Feelings such as boredom, sadness, or even joy/celebration
- Poor macronutrient balance—too low in protein or fat or too high or low in carbohydrates
- Lack of fiber
- Habit—our palate is trained to expect it
- Poor blood glucose control
- Monthly hormonal fluctuations, PMS, etc.
- Nutrient-poor diet (lack of the nutrition our body needs)
- Hormonal dysregulation, HPA axis dysfunction, "adrenal fatigue"

So, what does that mean for you? You're probably wondering WHAT TO DO when cravings hit during the program. First of all, be kind to yourself. We're looking to nourish and support our bodies, not to fight them. So, if you give in to a little something, then just get past it: move on and reset. Don't give up!

But, to help you avoid craving as much as possible, here are some tips:

- Be patient. Well-designed ancestral diets help with cravings AFTER a period of adjustment. There is usually a period of withdrawal from high-glycemic carbohydrates (i.e., sugar, refined flour) and artificial sweeteners, then a period of craving them MUCH less. So, hang in there!
- Avoid artificial sweeteners. They prevent the palate from adjusting to a less sweet diet. They also have been shown to have negative effects on blood glucose and the microbiome.
- Get enough sleep. Try to be in bed at least eight hours per night.
- Have a daily stress-reduction technique: meditation, gentle exercise such as yoga, coloring, etc.
- Drink water, sparkling water, or herbal tea with EVERY meal and snack. If you don't like the flavor of water, then try keeping a pitcher in the fridge with some lemon, lime, or cucumber slices in it.
- Avoid stocking tempting foods around your house, especially during the twenty-one days.
- When a craving hits you anyway, try a cup of tea, a walk, getting busy with a project, playing with your kids, or cleaning house. Avoid turning to TV, email, phone, Facebook (screens) during this time.
- Imagine your end goal. How do you want to look and feel at the end of the twenty-one days? Close your eyes and actually visualize it. Think of all the hard work you've done to support yourself—planning, cooking, etc. You deserve to be and feel well! Sometimes putting that craving into perspective helps to make it go away.

There are dietary supplements that can help. However, no supplement can fix a lack of sleep, under-hydration, or good hormone regulation on its own. So, I recommend doing your best, with the right mind-set in place. Remember: you are a person of infinite value and worth. We all crave a treat now and then. Don't ever let that fact make you feel bad about yourself.

4. Self-Acceptance

So, hang with me on this. I got a PR (personal record/best) for "the clean and jerk" the other day: 132 lbs, or 60 kg. I'm a fairly small person, so some may think it's pretty amazing that I can get that amount of weight over my head in a matter of seconds. Or those who are actually good at Olympic lifting might consider it closer to their warm-up weight. Either way, I don't care. Whatever you can do, *I think it's awesome*. My own lifting is about me—I don't compare. Because comparing makes us crazy. When we get jealous of someone else, we're in a negative place. When we enjoy doing better than someone else, we're in a negative place. Unfortunately, that's where the world tries to put us. I'm talking about the Photoshopped woman on the magazine cover in the checkout line. The video on your Facebook feed of a nine-months-pregnant woman lifting heavier weights than you. The "Summer Is Coming" email you open to see a perfect body in a bikini.

Forget that noise. You're on an amazing path. Keep track of your progress. Stay focused. Worry about getting a "PR" for your own wellness, not meeting some insane, unreachable standard.

I know: easier said than done. It's a process, but growing self-acceptance is *critical* for happiness and wellness. Here are a few things that can help:

- Think of something that makes you feel happy and that you're good at. Make more time for that.
- Surround yourself with positive, life-giving people. Set boundaries with the others.
- Stop keeping magazines around the house that lead to negative self-talk.
- Take social media fasts.
- That email makes you feel yucky? Unsubscribe.
- Check out the "Body Confidence" scene. There's a pretty good, free ten-day series here: http://summerinnanen.com/

In short, keep in mind your immense worth. Nothing that makes you doubt it is worth your time. Don't let anything make you feel like you need to beat yourself up over not having the perfect diet or the perfect body. Stress and self-loathing are pretty toxic. I find that when self-acceptance improves, wellness usually does so as well.

12

Continuing the Bone Broth Lifestyle

The most common question I get from my program participants is: "What do I do after this ends?!?" Bone broth, ancestral foods, and intermittent fasting can be a sustainable, enjoyable lifestyle choice going forward. In fact, I would argue that they really are essential for optimal wellness. However, although it's nice to have everything laid out for twenty-one days, both ancestral diets and intermittent fasting should eventually become individualized.

The "right" diet actually depends on the person—no two of my clients end up with the same recommendation. Energy needs and preferences vary. Some people can get away with more gray area foods than others, and some can even consume small amounts of completely Neolithic foods without issue. On the other hand, some people need therapeutic diets to fully feel well. Macronutrient balance is another highly individual factor; some people need much more carbohydrates than others, and our genetic makeup even impacts our carbohydrate needs.

With regard to fasting, most people go through periods where it is more appropriate than others. During a time that you are sleep-deprived or very stressed, it may be a good idea to fast less, if at all. When you are rested and pursuing a health goal, that is a time when it may help to fast more consistently.

Even bone broth may be a better fit at some times more than others. I recommend trying to consume one cup most days for general wellness and three cups per day if you're using it to address a disease or injury. Yet, you may sometimes be busy or traveling, and bone broth may not fit during those times. It could be detrimental to stress out over bone broth when it just isn't practical.

Bottom line, stress is extremely harmful. So, it's not helpful to constantly worry about creating the perfect diet, eating pattern, and ancestral lifestyle. Practice self-acceptance and work toward the best fit that you can make for your personal situation and preferences.

All that being said, there are times when a more targeted approach is needed. Some diseases and conditions require dietary and treatment plans that go beyond the scope of this book. Some of them will actually not be resolved with even the most perfect diet and lifestyle; additional types of treatment may be required. In these cases, working with a professional can be extremely helpful.

To summarize Robb Wolf, the ultimate test is how we look, feel, and perform. I recommend following the twenty-one-day program in this book, then using the Resources section (see page 192) to start experimenting yourself. Bottom line, if you aren't able to experience improvements in the way you look, feel, and perform, it might be time to get help. I have provided some ways to find functional and ancestral medicine practitioners in the Resources section toward the end of this book (see page 192).

My genuine hope is that this book has benefited you. It is truly amazing what a difference an ancestral approach can make. Unfortunately, we live in a world where dietary advice is often confusing, conflicting, and sometimes even harmful. This comes at a time when nutrition-related disease is at an all-time high and is only increasing in incidence. You now have the knowledge of what dietary approach is truly healthful. Unfortunately, your friends and family are not likely to get this knowledge from their healthcare provider or from a public health message. Thus, I encourage you to share this precious truth with them. I wish you and yours all the best in health and wellness.

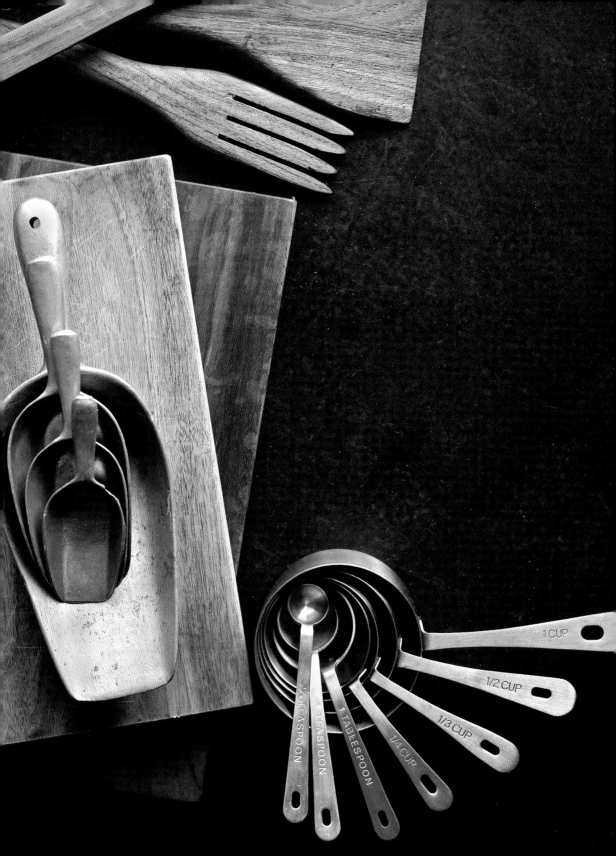

13

Recipes

Bone Broth Tutorial

Read over this tutorial before you make your first batch of bone broth, so that you're ready to rock. It shows a combination of beef and chicken broth. You basically follow the same steps as any kind of broth, but with different cooking times. Here we go!

1. Place bones, vinegar, and water in large stock pot, using enough filtered water to cover the bones. Alternately, (if yours is large enough) you may use a slow cooker on Low. If using a slow cooker, you can add all the veggies/herbs at the beginning.
2. Let your broth sit for 30–60 minutes before turning on the heat if possible (omit this step if using slow cooker).
3. Heat the pot, covered, on high. Bring to a boil, then uncover and turn down heat to low (a gentle simmer). Scoop off any scum from the top. I find that quality bones have little or no scum, so don't worry if you don't see any.

NOTE

If you follow a low-FODMAP diet or have food sensitivities, you may omit any vegetables or herbs desired.

4. Add all vegetables and herbs (if you haven't done so already).
5. Place the lid slightly askew and cook on low for 12–24 hours, periodically skimming any scum from the top. Add water as needed to keep the contents covered. IMPORTANT: If you're cooking meat (i.e. a roast or whole chicken) with your broth, make sure to remove it around the 6–8 hour point. Save the meat for your meals, and return the bones to the broth to keep cooking.
6. Remove all of the large solids with tongs or a slotted spoon, saving bones and any remaining meat. You may refrigerate any meat for meals and re-use the bones up to two more times for broth. *Extra credit: If you get any marrow from the bones, eat it with a little salt.*
7. Filter the remaining broth with a fine mesh strainer. Discard filtered solids and refrigerate broth in glass containers.

8. Once the broth is chilled, remove the fat layer from the top (you can save it for later cooking use).
9. Season broth as needed for drinking or cooking. Never boil it when re-heating.
10. Store your broth in the refrigerator up to one week or in the freezer for up to three months. Many experienced broth-ers freeze it in small containers or ice cube trays so that they can easily throw it into their cooking on a regular basis.

NOTE
Ideally your broth will have a gelatinous texture when it's cold. Don't worry either way.

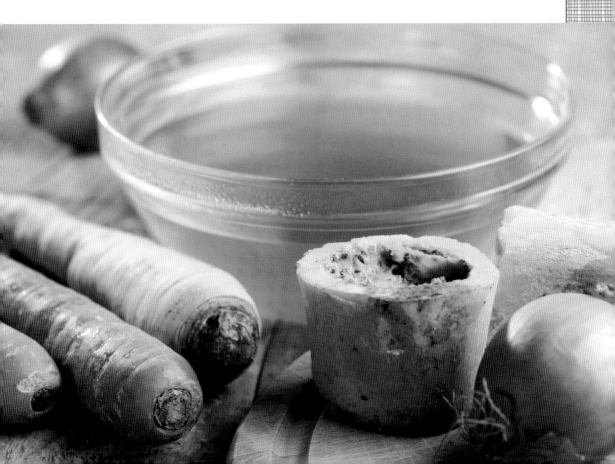

Broths

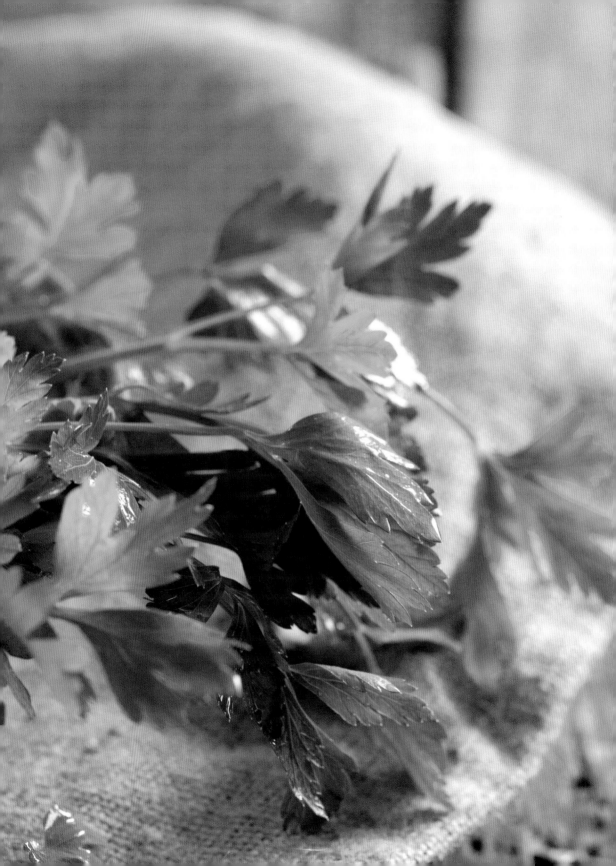

Whole Chicken Broth

Have your chicken (bone broth) and eat it too! This recipe makes both cooked chicken and bone broth. The longer you cook it, the more nutritious the broth will be. Work the timing around your schedule and when you need the broth for breakfast, snacks, recipes, etc. If this is your *first* bone broth (wee!) then take a deep breath and get in there. You'll be cranking out batches of goodness with ease in no time.

Prep time: 10 min / Cook time: 10–18 hours / Total time: 10–18 hours

Ingredients

1 whole organic chicken, 3–4 pounds (½–2 kg)
¼ cup (60 ml) apple cider vinegar
1 white or yellow onion, peeled and roughly chopped
3 whole cloves garlic, peeled
2 carrots, peeled and roughly chopped
2 celery stalks, roughly chopped
2 bay leaves
2 sprigs fresh thyme
2 sprigs fresh parsley
½ teaspoon ground black pepper, or to taste
Filtered water (amount needed to cover, ~3–4 qt/L)

NOTE
If you are eating a low-FODMAP diet or have food sensitivities, you may omit any vegetables or herbs desired.

Instructions

1. Check inside chicken for any plastic bags. Remove the bag(s), retrieve any giblets, and use them in the recipe.
2. Place all ingredients in slow cooker, using enough filtered water to cover the chicken. It's okay if you just *nearly* cover it—it will shrink down. You need to be able to cover it with a lid. Alternately, you may cook on very low heat (barely

Continued on next page.

simmering) on stovetop in a large stock pot (use smallest burner on lowest heat).

3. Cover and cook on low for 10–18 hours, periodically skimming any scum from the top. Add water as needed to keep contents covered. Do not boil.

4. To prevent dry chicken: Remove whole chicken around the 7–8 hour point and let cool. Remove meat from bones and set aside. Place bones back in broth and continue cooking. (Removing the chicken meat now will prevent it from becoming tough and dry. You won't be using it any longer for this recipe, so you may refrigerate it for use in future meals.)

5. When broth is done cooking, turn off heat and cool slightly. Remove all solids with tongs or a slotted spoon, saving the bones. (You may re-use bones up to two more times for broth.)

6. Filter remaining broth with a fine mesh strainer. Discard filtered solids and refrigerate broth in glass container(s).

7. Once broth is chilled, remove fat layer from the top (may save for cooking use).

8. Salt broth as needed for cooking and drinking. Never boil when re-heating.

9. Store in glass containers in refrigerator up to one week or in freezer up to three months.

Makes 4 servings chicken (all vegetables and herbs strained and removed)
1 serving = 196 calories, 5 g fat, 35 g protein, 0 g carbohydrates, 0 g fiber

Makes variable servings broth (serving size: 1 cup/8 oz/240 ml)
1 serving = 28 calories, 0.5 g fat, 6 g protein, 0 g carbohydrates, 0 g fiber

Legit Beef Bone Broth

Not scary. You're the boss. Show those bones what a caveperson you are—and reap the wellness benefits. The longer you cook this, the more nutritious the broth will be. Work the timing around your schedule and when you'll need the broth for breakfast, snacks, recipes, etc. I prefer a slow cooker for this recipe so that I can leave it going overnight, but stovetop works great as well.

Prep time: 15 min / Cook time: 12–24 hours / Total time: 12–24 hours

Ingredients

4–6 pounds (2–3 kg) grass-fed beef bones
¼ cup (60 ml) apple cider vinegar
Filtered water (amount needed to cover all
    ingredients, ~4–5 qt/L)
1 onion, peeled and roughly chopped
3 whole cloves garlic, peeled
3 carrots, peeled and roughly chopped
3 celery stalks, roughly chopped
2 bay leaves
2 sprigs fresh thyme
2 sprigs fresh parsley
Black pepper to taste

NOTE

It's best if about half of the bones are marrow and/or knucklebones and the other half are meaty bones like short ribs and/or beef shanks. Don't stress over this though; get what you can.

Instructions

1. Place bones, vinegar, and water in large stock pot, using enough filtered water to cover the bones. Alternatively, (if yours is large enough) you may use a slow cooker on Low.
2. Let sit 30–60 minutes before turning on heat if possible (omit this step if using slow cooker).

NOTE

If you are eating a low-FODMAP diet or have food sensitivities, you may omit any vegetables or herbs desired.

Continued on next page.

3. Heat pot covered on high, bring to a boil, then uncover and turn down heat to low (a gentle simmer). Scoop off any scum from the top.
4. Add all remaining ingredients to the broth.
5. Add the lid slightly askew (small opening) and cook on low for 12–24 hours, periodically skimming any scum from the top. Add water as needed to keep contents covered.
6. Remove all solids with tongs or a slotted spoon, saving bones and meat. You may refrigerate the meat for meals and re-use the bones up to two more times for broth. *Extra credit: If you get any marrow from the bones, eat it with a little salt.*
7. Filter remaining broth with a fine mesh strainer. Discard filtered solids and refrigerate broth in glass containers.
8. Once broth is chilled, remove fat layer from the top (may save for cooking use).
9. Season broth as needed for drinking/cooking. Never boil when re-heating.
10. Store in glass containers in refrigerator up to one week or in freezer up to three months.

Makes variable servings broth (serving size: 1 cup/8 oz/240 ml)
1 serving = 28 calories, 0.5 g fat, 6 g protein, 0 g carbohydrates, 0 g fiber

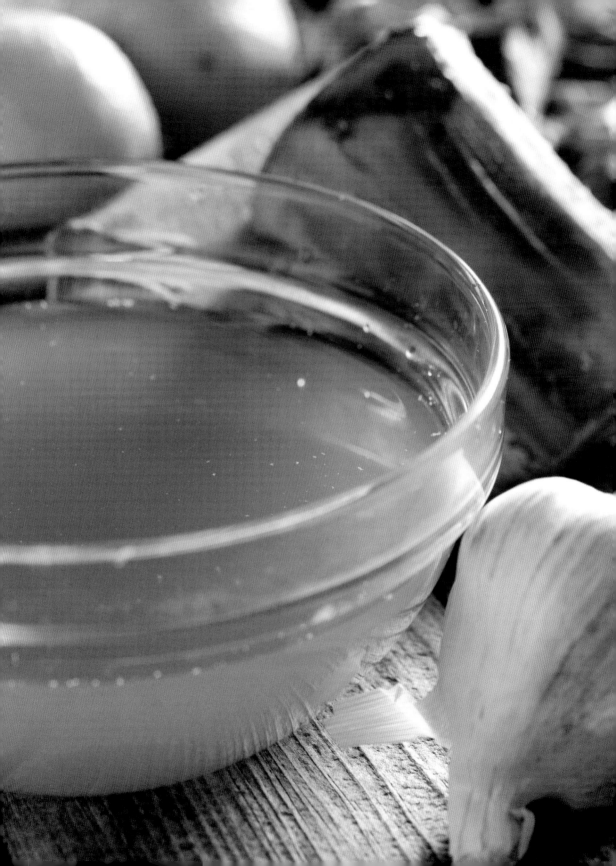

A Little Something Broth

There's a little something in there. It's like a sassier version of beef broth. You only go around once, so why not? If you know you don't like allspice, no problem—just leave it out. Or choose one of the million substitutions I listed.

Prep time: 15 min / Cook time: 12–24 hours / Total time: 12–24 hours

Ingredients
4–6 pounds (2–3 kg) grass-fed beef bones
¼ cup (60 ml) apple cider vinegar
Filtered water (amount needed to cover all
    ingredients, ~4–5 qt/L)
1 onion, peeled and roughly chopped
3 whole cloves garlic, peeled
3 carrots, peeled and roughly chopped
3 celery stalks, roughly chopped
2 bay leaves
2 sprigs fresh thyme
2 sprigs fresh parsley
Black pepper to taste
3 whole allspice berries, *or* ½ teaspoon ground allspice,
    or ½ teaspoon ground cinnamon + ⅛ teaspoon ground cloves,
    or 3 whole cloves

NOTE

It's best if about half of the bones are marrow and/or knucklebones and the other half are meaty bones like short ribs and/or beef shanks. Don't stress over this though; get what you can.

Instructions
1. Place bones, vinegar, and water in large stock pot, using enough filtered water to cover the bones. Alternatively, (if yours is large enough) you may use a slow cooker on Low.
2. Let the broth sit 30–60 minutes before turning on the heat if possible (omit this step if using slow cooker).

NOTE

If you are eating a low-FODMAP diet or have food sensitivities, you may omit any vegetables or herbs desired.

3. Heat pot, covered, on high. Bring to a boil, then uncover and turn down heat to low (a gentle simmer). Scoop off any scum from the top.
4. Add all remaining ingredients to the broth.
5. Place the lid slightly askew and cook on low for 12–24 hours, periodically skimming any scum from the top. Add water as needed to keep contents covered.
6. Remove all solids with tongs or a slotted spoon, saving bones and meat. You may refrigerate the meat for meals and re-use the bones up to two more times for broth. *Extra credit: If you get any marrow from the bones, eat it with a little salt.*
7. Filter remaining broth with a fine mesh strainer. Discard filtered solids and refrigerate broth in glass containers.
8. Once broth is chilled, remove fat layer from the top (may save for cooking use).
9. Season broth as needed for drinking/cooking. Never boil when re-heating.
10. Store in glass containers in refrigerator up to one week or in freezer up to three months.

Makes variable servings broth (serving size: 1 cup/8 oz/240 ml)
1 serving = 28 calories, 0.5 g fat, 6 g protein, 0 g carbohydrates, 0 g fiber

Inflammation-Fighting Broth

This recipe combines the benefits of bone broth with the anti-inflammatory properties of curcumin (found in turmeric) and garlic. Your body will say, "Thank you!" The longer you cook it, the more nutritious the broth will be. Work the timing around your schedule and when you'll need the broth for breakfast, snacks, recipes, etc.

Prep time: 10 min / Cook time: 12–24 hours / Total time: 12–24 hours

Ingredients

~4 pounds (2 kg) free-range chicken bones
¼ cup apple cider vinegar
1 large onion, peeled and chopped in quarters
6 cloves peeled garlic
2 teaspoons ground turmeric
1 bay leaf
Filtered water (amount needed to cover all ingredients, ~4–6 qt/L)

Instructions

1. Place all ingredients in a slow cooker, making sure you have enough filtered water to cover the chicken. Alternatively, you may cook on very low heat (barely simmering) on stovetop in large stock pot.
2. Cover and cook on Low for 12–24 hours, periodically skimming any scum from the top. Add water as need to keep contents covered.
3. Remove all solids with tongs or a slotted spoon, saving bones. You may re-use the bones up to two more times for broth. Filter remaining broth with a fine mesh strainer. Discard filtered solids and refrigerate broth in glass containers.

NOTE
If you are eating a low-FODMAP diet or have food sensitivities, you may omit any vegetables or herbs desired.

4. Once broth is chilled, remove fat layer from the top (save for cooking use). Store broth in glass containers in refrigerator up to one week or freezer up to three months. Never boil when re-heating.

Makes variable servings broth (serving size: 1 cup/8 oz/240 ml)
1 serving = 28 calories, 0.5 g fat, 6 g protein, 0 g carbohydrates, 0 g fiber

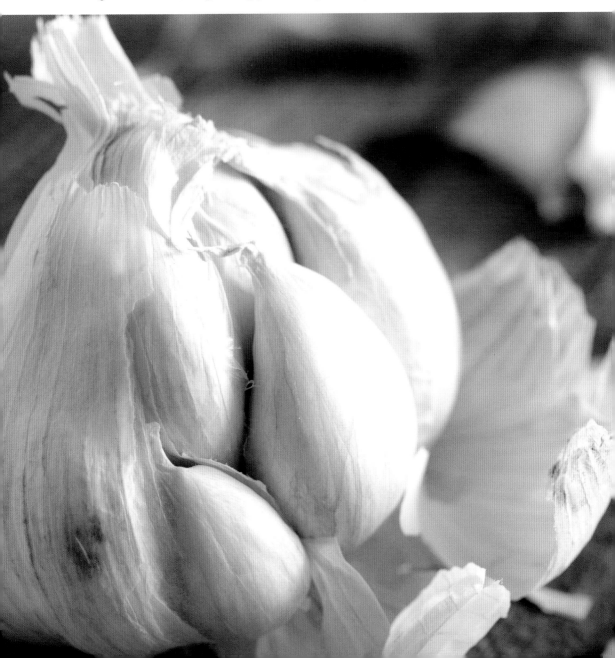

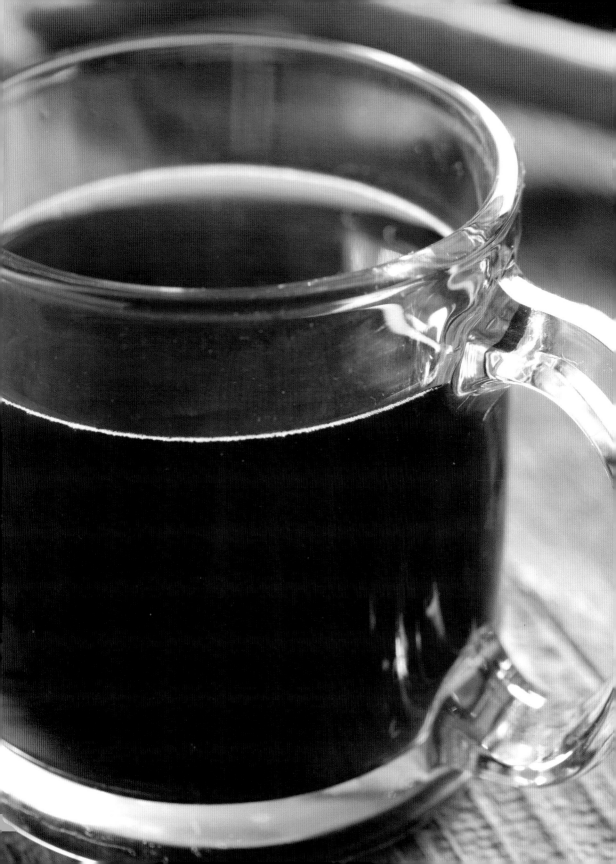

Drink Your Broth and Eat It Too

So, I can make bone broth and also have meat ready for dinner at the same time? Yes, please. This mama is busy. I'm sure you are too. If you can't find beef shanks, then use beef bones and throw a tough beef roast in there. You're basically "slow braising" it.

Prep time: 15 min / Cook time: 6–12 hours / Total time: 6–12 hours

Ingredients

4–6 pounds (2–3 kg) grass-fed beef shanks
¼ cup apple cider vinegar
Filtered water to cover all ingredients (~4–5 qt)
3 whole cloves garlic, peeled
1 onion, peeled and roughly chopped
3 carrots, peeled and roughly chopped
3 celery stalks, roughly chopped
2 bay leaves
2 sprigs fresh thyme
2 sprigs fresh rosemary
1 piece peeled ginger, about 1"
1 teaspoon ground turmeric, *or* 1"–2" peeled root
1½ teaspoon sea salt
Black pepper to taste

NOTE
Alternatively, use a tough beef roast (2–4 lbs/1–2 kg) with beef bones (~4 lbs/2 kg).

NOTE
If you are eating a low-FODMAP diet or have food sensitivities, you may omit any vegetables or herbs desired.

Instructions

1. Place beef shanks (or roast and bones), vinegar, and water in large stock pot, using enough filtered water to cover the bones. Alternatively, (if yours is large enough) you may use a slow cooker on Low.
2. Heat pot, covered, on high. Bring to a boil, then uncover and turn down heat to low (a gentle simmer). Scoop off any scum from the top.
3. Add all remaining ingredients to the broth.

Continued on next page.

4. Place the lid slightly askew and cook on low for 6–12 hours, periodically skimming any scum from the top. Add water as needed to keep contents covered.
5. Remove all solids with tongs or a slotted spoon, saving bones and meat. You may refrigerate the meat for meals and re-use the bones up to two more times for broth—or keep the bones cooking longer if you like. *Extra credit: If you get any marrow from the bones, eat it with a little salt.*
6. Filter remaining broth with a fine mesh strainer. Discard filtered solids and refrigerate broth in glass containers.
7. Once broth is chilled, remove fat layer from the top (may save for cooking use).
8. Season broth as needed for drinking/cooking. Never boil when re-heating.
9. Store in glass containers in refrigerator up to one week or in freezer up to three months.

Makes variable beef servings (1 serving = 3 oz cooked meat)
1 serving = 171 calories, 5 g fat, 29 g protein, 0 g carbohydrates, 0 g fiber

Makes variable broth servings (1 serving = 1 cup/8 oz/240 ml without fat)
1 serving = 28 calories, 0.5 g fat, 6 g protein, 0 g carbohydrates, 0 g fiber

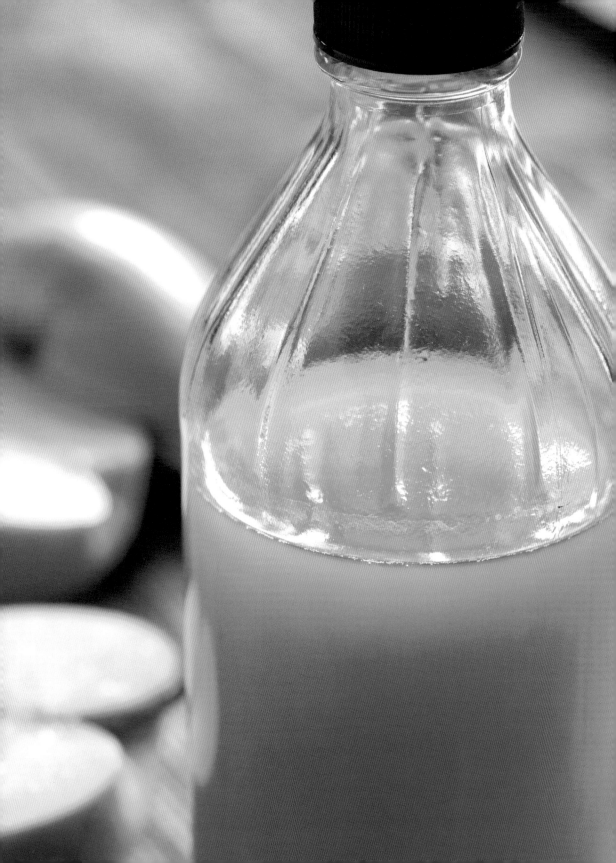

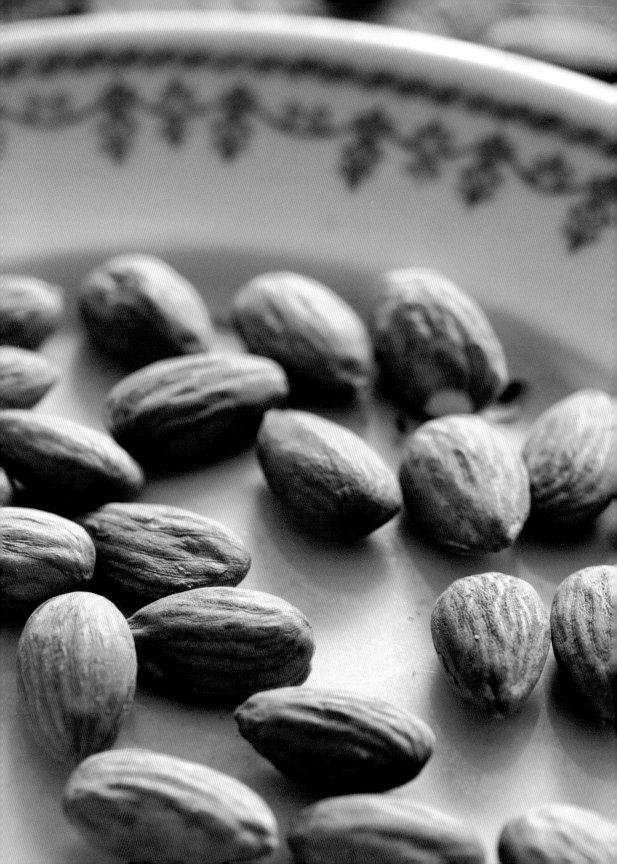

Snacks

Note:
Besides these recipes, most of the program's
snacks are just small servings of foods like
hard-boiled eggs, nuts, or seeds. For more
details, see Meal Plans, starting on page 77.

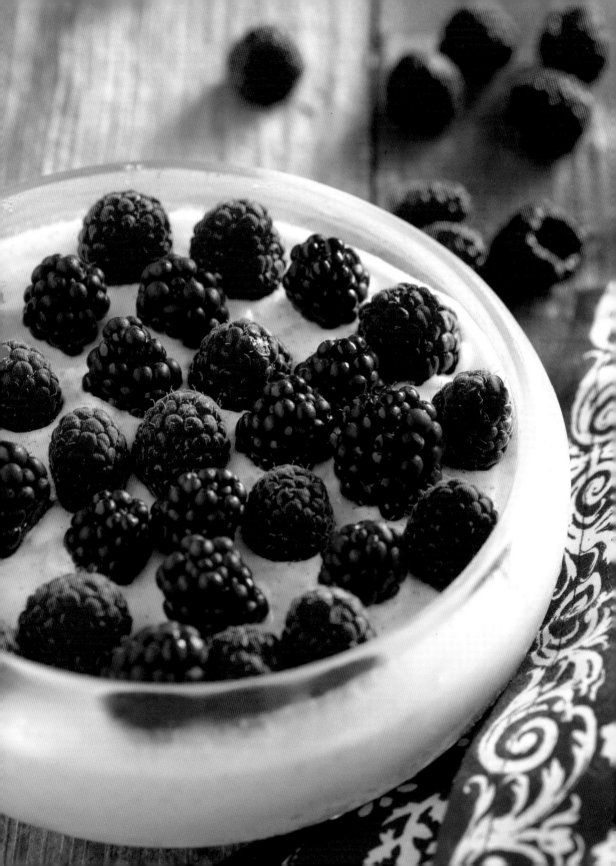

#SoGood Chia Pudding

I try not to be one of those people. You know: constant social media feed of their amazing food. Amazing vacation. Amazing everything. Whatever. But really, eating this way does make me feel pretty awesome. Every time I eat this pudding, I get *so* tempted to Instagram a picture just to rub it in. #SoGood doesn't even do it justice, really.

Prep time: 5 min / Total time: 2 hours

Ingredients

1 can (~14 oz) full-fat coconut milk (chilled if possible)
2 Tablespoons (30 ml) honey or maple syrup
1 teaspoon (5 ml) real vanilla extract
¼ teaspoon (1 ml) cinnamon
¼ teaspoon (1 ml) ground cardamom (optional)
⅛ teaspoon (.5 ml) sea salt
¼ cup (60 ml) whole chia seeds
Unsweetened coconut flakes (optional garnish)
Berries (optional garnish)
Crushed nuts (optional garnish)

Instructions

1. Blend all ingredients except the chia seeds in a blender (don't skip this step or you will get gross clumps).
2. Slowly add the chia seeds to your mixture while whisking (not blending) constantly to break up clumps.
3. Divide into serving bowls if desired. Put it all in the fridge for 2 hours. Ideally, try to mix it a few times during this period to make sure no clumps form.
4. If desired, garnish with coconut flakes, berries, or crushed nuts. Yum!

Makes 5 servings
1 serving (without garnish) = 241 calories, 4 g protein, 14 g carbohydrates, 21 g fat, 5 g fiber

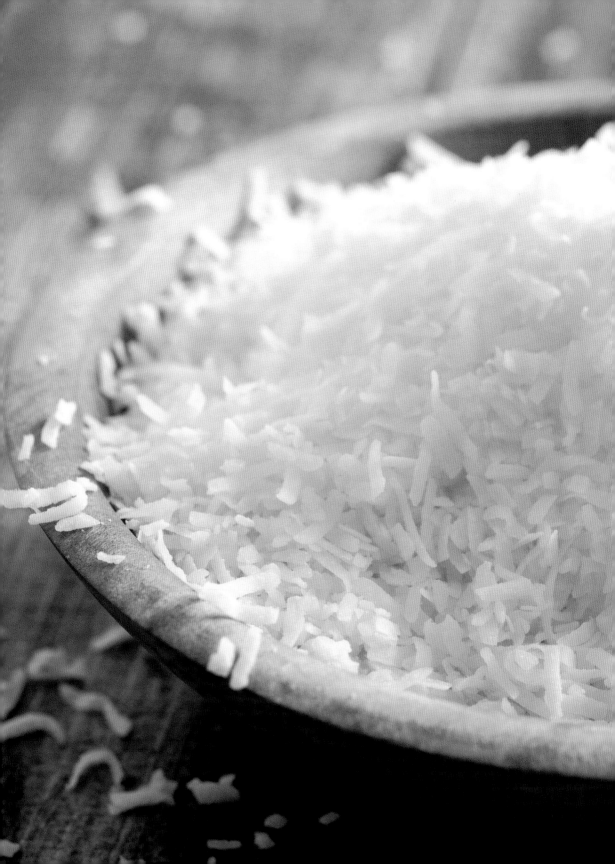

Chocolate Coconut Balls

When all else fails, chocolate. When chocolate can be a snack that is packed with healthy MCT oil and low in carbs? Even less reason to say "no." If you have trouble sourcing the coconut butter and unsweetened coconut locally, there are many options online.

Prep time: 10 min / Cooking time: 15–30 min / Total time: 25–40 min

Ingredients

½ cup (120 ml) coconut butter (also known as creamed coconut, coconut cream concentrate, or coconut manna—NOT coconut oil or coconut milk)
½ cup (120 ml) unsweetened shredded coconut
1 Tablespoon (15 ml) raw honey
1 Tablespoon (15 ml) cocoa powder (optional)
1 teaspoon (5 ml) real vanilla extract, or to taste

NOTE
Make sure to watch these closely in the oven—they're good a little undercooked.

Instructions

1. Preheat oven to 350°F. Mix coconut butter, shredded coconut, honey, cocoa powder, and vanilla together in a large bowl.
2. Form 12 balls using about 1–2 Tablespoons (15–30 ml) of the mixture for each. If the mixture is too runny, refrigerate it for 15–30 minutes.
3. Place the coconut balls on a lined baking sheet.
4. Bake at 350°F (180°C) for 8–10 minutes until fragrant and slightly golden (watch carefully).
5. Let cool completely before eating and store in the refrigerator.

Makes 4 servings (1 serving = 3 balls)
1 serving = 184 calories, 17 g fat, 2 g protein, 10 g carbohydrates, 3 g fiber

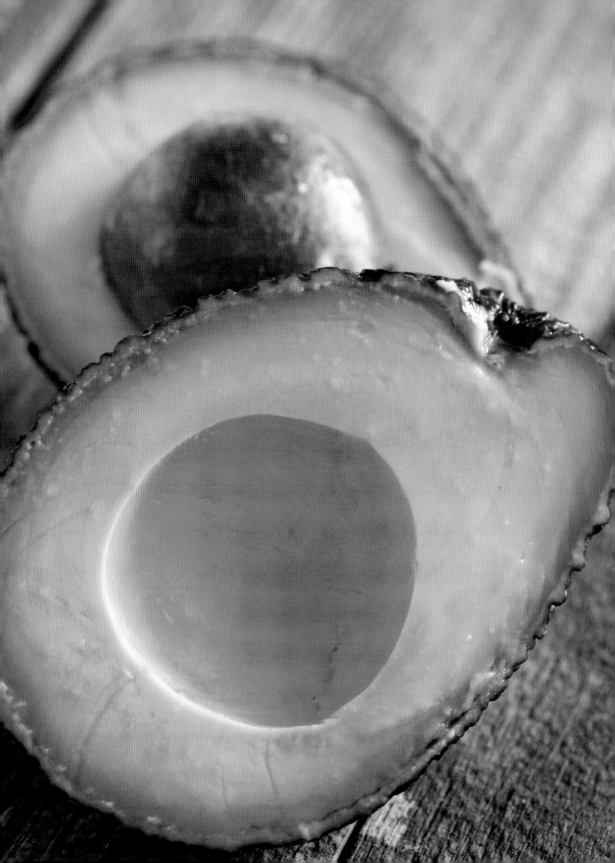

Avocado To Go

Avocados may be one of the most perfect foods, but they're not doing you any good getting over-ripe on your kitchen counter. This is a great way to use them up quickly without a lot of fuss and to get an incredibly nourishing snack while you're at it. If you're in a rush, just throw this in a bowl and eat it on the go!

Prep time: 5 min / Total time: 5 min

Ingredients
½ avocado
1 medium vine-ripe tomato
1 teaspoon (5 ml) olive oil
Sea salt to taste

Instructions
1. Peel and de-seed the avocado, then roughly chop half of it.
2. Roughly chop your tomato.
3. Combine chopped avocado and tomato, olive oil, and sea salt to taste. May add pepper and/or additional spices as desired.

Makes 1 serving
1 serving = 256 calories, 20 g fat, 5 g protein, 17 g carbohydrates, 10 g fiber

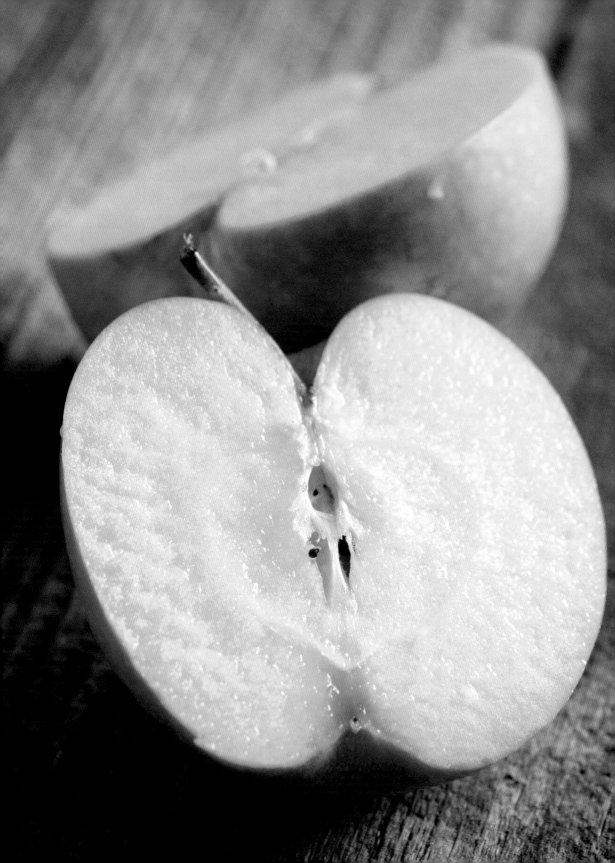

Breakfast

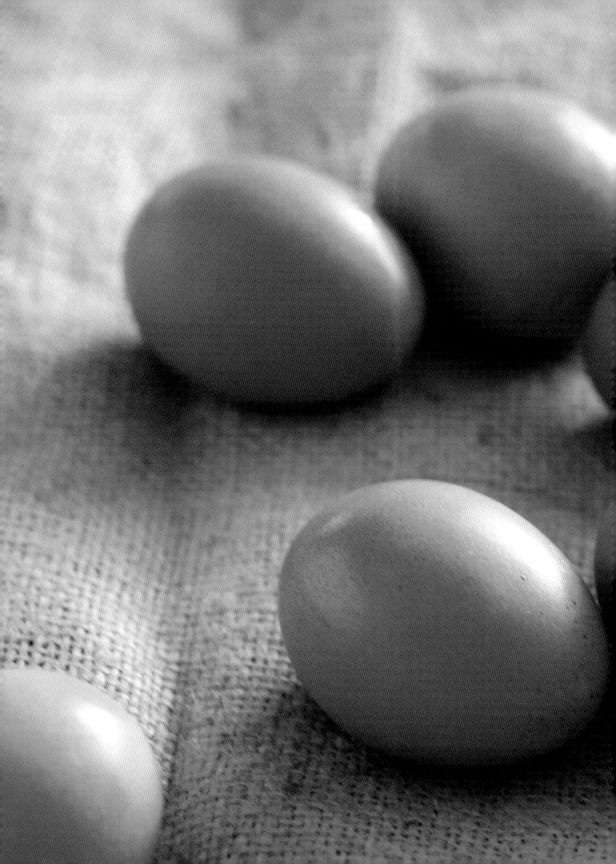

Veg & Eggs

Good morning and welcome to the perfect low-carb breakfast. Or dinner. Or snack. OK, this meal just kind of happens whenever I need some food and have no leftovers. You can really use this as a template and throw in any greens and/or leftover veggies you have. Got some ham or smoked salmon around? Hit that. Fat + egg + veg = amazing.

Prep time: 10 min / Cook time: 10 min / Total time: 10 min

Ingredients
1 teaspoon (5 ml) coconut oil
1 cup loose baby spinach
2 organic, free-range eggs
Sea salt and freshly ground pepper to taste
½ avocado, thinly sliced

Instructions
1. Heat the coconut oil in a small saucepan over medium heat.
2. Once hot, sauté the spinach until it is cooked down and wilted.
3. Meanwhile, whisk the eggs, salt, and pepper in a bowl. Make sure to whisk enough to fully combine the eggs and get them a little lighter and frothy.
4. Pour the eggs over the spinach and cook/scramble them gently.
5. Transfer the eggs to a plate and top them with the thinly sliced avocado.

Makes 1 serving
1 serving = 354 calories, 28 g fat, 15 g protein, 14 g carbohydrates, 9 g fiber

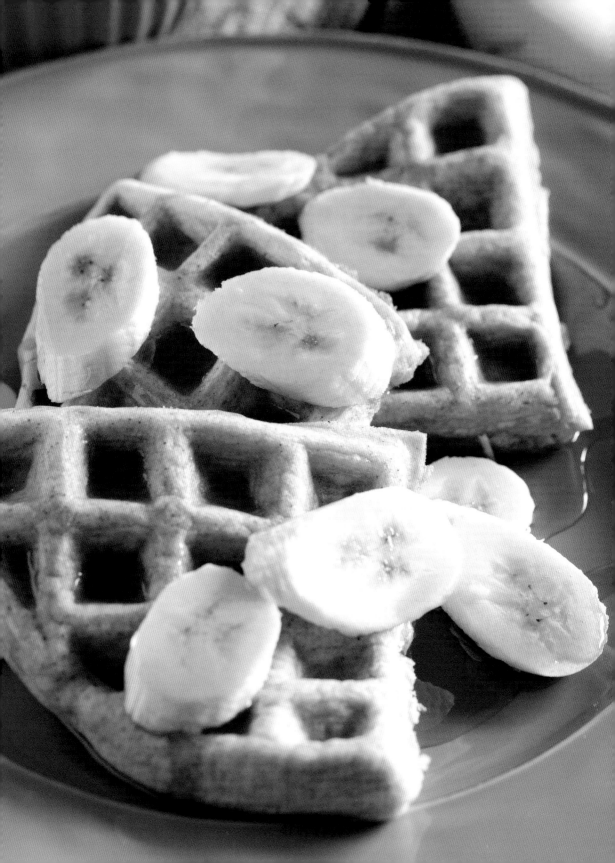

Grain-Free Waffles

This is the holy grail, people. Not only do these waffles cook up quickly and taste amazing, but they don't contain a bunch of grain-free "flour." This means you get a good dose of clean protein and fat without a huge amount of carbs or inflammatory fats. During the twenty-one days, I recommend topping them with a little nut butter. Later, you can experiment with the other toppings listed below, or try adding carob chips or a chopped apple to the mixture.

Prep time: 15 min / Total time: 15 min

Ingredients

6 eggs
1 ripe banana, mashed
½ teaspoon (2½ ml) baking powder
½ teaspoon (2½ ml) sea salt
⅓ cup (80 ml) coconut flour
¼ teaspoon (1 ml) cinnamon
4 Tablespoons (60 ml) coconut oil (melted)

ALTERNATIVE
This batter recipe also works for pancakes!

Instructions

1. Preheat your waffle iron.
2. Whisk the eggs in a medium bowl.
3. Add the mashed banana, baking powder, sea salt, coconut flour, and cinnamon and mix well.
4. Add the melted coconut oil and mix again.
5. Cook your batter in the waffle iron, using ~⅓ cup batter per waffle.
6. Serve with your topping of choice.

TOPPINGS
A few of my family's favorite toppings are: nut butter, pure fruit preserves, maple syrup, coconut whipped cream, pan-fried apples, or a little honey.

Makes 4 servings
1 serving (no topping) = 308 calories, 11 g protein, 14 g carbohydrates, 23 g fat, 4 g fiber

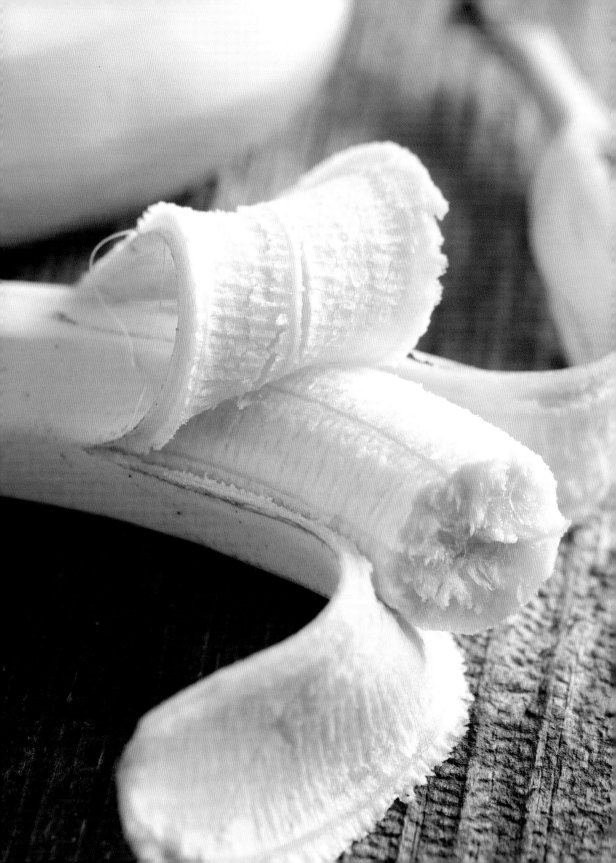

Banana Pancakes

A common way that "ancestral diets" can go wrong is the overuse of nut and coconut flours to re-create baked goods. It's fun to occasionally try a paleo baking recipe but I wouldn't be making almond flour pancakes for breakfast on the daily. But still—we need pancakes. This version is made of mostly eggs and bananas: protein, fat, carbs, check! A great breakfast, dinner, snack, anytime food. Make sure to keep them small so that they're easy to flip.

Prep time: 10 min / Cook time: 15 min / Total time: 25 min

Ingredients

1½ ripe bananas
2 eggs
⅛ teaspoon (½ ml) baking powder
½ teaspoon (2½ ml) cinnamon
¼ teaspoon (1 ml) real vanilla extract
½ Tablespoon (7½ ml) coconut oil

Instructions

1. Coarsely mash the bananas in a medium-sized bowl with a fork. Add all other ingredients except the coconut oil and combine well.
2. Heat coconut oil in skillet or large pan on the stove over medium heat.
3. Pour just ~2 Tablespoons batter per pancake onto hot pan/skillet (make minis). This makes it easier to flip the pancakes. Cook ~3 minutes, or until lightly browned on bottom.
4. Flip pancakes and cook ~2 minutes, or until lightly browned. If pancakes flip fairly easily, you can make them larger the next time you fill pan.
5. Serve with topping of choice!

Makes 1 serving
1 serving = 370 calories, 17 g fat, 14 g protein, 41 g carbohydrates, 5 g fiber

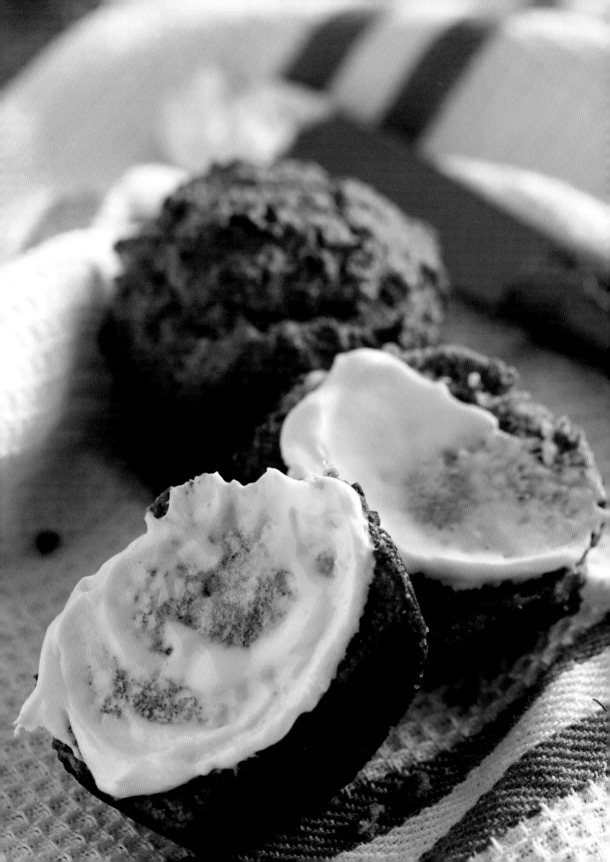

Keeper Muffins

I've had my fair share of paleo baking disasters. For some reason, it can be hard to nail it. For that reason, I really treasure a quality paleo baking recipe. We all need a good muffin option, right? You can swap out the apple for berries or fruit if you like. Eat one for a snack or two for breakfast. Oh, and be careful to take these puppies out of the oven *before* they dry out!

Prep time: 10 min / Cook time: 30 min / Total time: 40 min

Ingredients

1 cup (240 ml) almond flour
3 Tablespoons (45 ml) coconut flour
1 Tablespoon (15 ml) cinnamon (or pumpkin pie spice)
½ teaspoon (2½ ml) baking soda
⅛ (1 ml) teaspoon sea salt

3 large eggs, whisked
¼ cup (60 ml) coconut oil, melted
2 Tablespoons (30 ml) raw honey
1 very ripe banana, mashed
1 medium apple (or 2 small), cored and diced

Instructions

1. Preheat oven to 350°F (170°C).
2. Place muffin liners in 12 muffin tin cups (or lightly oil the cups).
3. In a large bowl, combine and mix almond flour, coconut flour, cinnamon, baking soda, and salt.
4. In a separate bowl, combine eggs, oil, honey, mashed banana, and diced apple. Mix thoroughly.
5. Combine your wet and dry mixtures and gently mix until just combined.
6. Distribute batter evenly among your muffin cups.
7. Bake for 20–25 minutes, checking/rotating halfway through, then every 5–10 minutes.
8. Remove muffins from the oven when a knife comes out nearly clean, being careful not to overcook.
9. Let muffins cool on a rack.

Makes 12 servings (1 serving = 1 muffin)
1 serving = 205 calories, 16 g fat, 6 g protein, 13 g carbohydrates, 4 g fiber

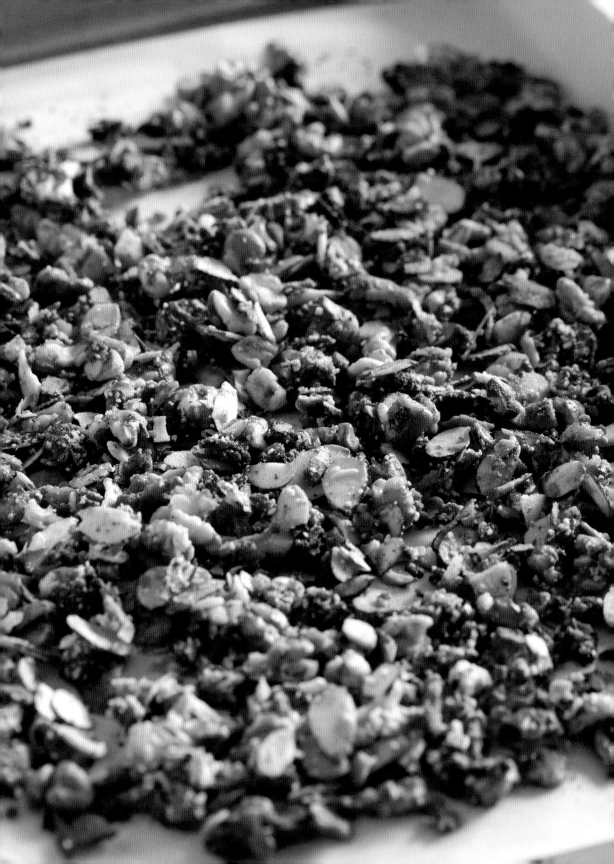

Kitchen Sink "Granola"

Do your crazy thing here. If you have some extra nuts, dried fruit, or seeds to get rid of, now is your big chance. You could also use honey instead of maple syrup or a different kind of spice. This might be good with a little nutmeg or cardamom. Got some citrus going bad? Throw in some zest and/or juice! When your family devours the final product, you can credit your own genius. *fist bump*

Prep time: 10 min / Cook time: 15 min / Total time: 25 min

Ingredients

1 cup (240 ml) sliced almonds
1 cup (240 ml) chopped walnuts
½ cup (120 ml) pitted dates, chopped
⅓ cup (80 ml) unsweetened shredded coconut
2 Tablespoons (30 ml) whole chia seeds

¼ cup (60 ml) blanched almond flour (meal)
¼ cup (60 ml) coconut oil, melted
2 Tablespoons (30 ml) maple syrup
2 teaspoons (10 ml) vanilla extract
1 teaspoon (5 ml) pumpkin pie spice (or ground cinnamon)
¼ teaspoon (1 ml) sea salt

Instructions

1. Preheat your oven to 350°F (170°C). Line a rimmed baking sheet with parchment paper or foil.
2. In a large bowl, combine and mix all ingredients together. Spread the mixture evenly on your prepared sheet.
3. Bake for 15 minutes, rotating halfway through, and checking every few minutes after the 10-minute mark.
4. Let cool completely before serving (let harden).

Makes 8 servings
1 serving = 358 calories, 27 g fat, 8 g protein, 25 g carbohydrates, 6 g fiber

Good Bugs Smoothie

Yes—delicious fermented foods! If you don't have access to kombucha, you may substitute 1 serving probiotic powder dissolved in ½ cup water or water kefir. If you tolerate dairy: kefir or organic, full-fat, plain yogurt are other possible substitutes. Worst case scenario: use extra almond milk instead.

Prep time: 5 min / Total time: 5 min

Ingredients
1 frozen banana
½ cup (120 ml) frozen mixed berries
½ cup (120 ml) unsweetened almond milk
½ cup (120 ml) kombucha (original or ginger flavor)
1 Tablespoon (15 ml) coconut oil

Instructions
1. Combine banana, frozen berries, almond milk, kombucha, and coconut oil in a blender. Add additional water as needed for texture.
2. Serve in a tall glass, maybe garnishing with fresh berries.

Makes 1 serving
1 serving = 311 calories, 16 g fat, 2 g protein, 46 g carbohydrates, 6 g fiber

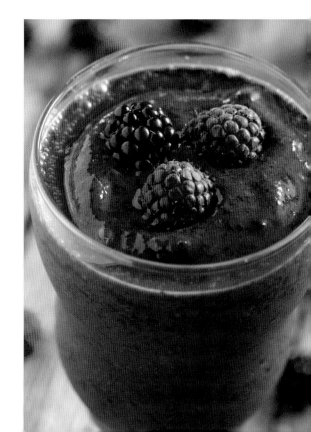

Wake Up Smoothie

Woke up ready to conquer the day? Or are you more in need of a way to wipe the slate clean? Either way, this smoothie is here to deliver. Fiber, protein, healthy fat, energy . . . it's all there. Even my kids love this smoothie, so I use it as a sneaky way to get some veggies in them. Feel free to experiment with some spices like cinnamon, ground ginger, or nutmeg. If you have a heavy workout ahead, why not throw in some nuts or avocado? Here's to a beautiful morning!

Prep time: 5 min / Total time: 5 min

Ingredients

¼ cup (60 ml) coconut milk

1 frozen banana

1 peeled carrot

2 peeled tangerines (or mandarin oranges), de-seeded

½ cup kale

1 Tablespoon (15 ml) chia seeds

¼ cup (60 ml) cold water, plus extra as needed for texture

Coconut flakes, *or* cinnamon (for garnish, optional)

Instructions

1. If you haven't done so already, thoroughly combine the contents of your can of coconut milk. Measure out the ¼ cup you need for the recipe. You may refrigerate the leftovers for up to one week or freeze them.
2. Combine banana, carrot, tangerines, kale, chia seeds, ¼ cup coconut milk, and ¼ cup water in a blender. Add a little more water as needed to reach desired consistency.
3. Serve in a tall glass and, if desired, garnish with coconut flakes or a sprinkle of cinnamon.

Makes 1 serving

1 serving = 346 calories, 15 g fat, 6 g protein, 50 g carbohydrates, 10 g fiber

Lunch and Dinner

Note:
Besides these recipes, most of
the program's lunches are dinner
leftovers. This just makes
life easier!

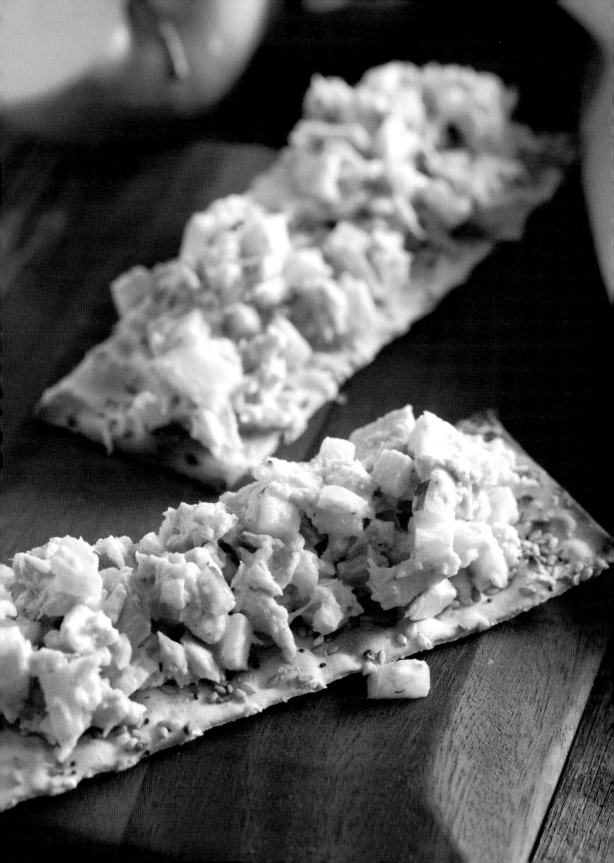

Curried Tuna Salad

The other day, I took my two- and four-year-old boys to an indoor playground. I brought this salad on a bed of spinach/cucumber/tomato for myself. I ordered kid's meals for the boys as a special treat. Before their meals arrived they had *completely* killed my whole meal—I got nothing! I often get the question, "How can I get my kids to eat healthy foods like fruits and vegetables?" Have them around. Eat them yourself. Make them in fun and interesting ways. Leave them laying around when your kids are hungry . . .

Prep time: 10 min / Cook time: none / Total time: 10 min

Ingredients
6 oz (170 g) canned tuna (packed in water)
1 medium tart apple
2 Tablespoons (30 ml) finely chopped red onion
2 Tablespoons (30 ml) finely chopped celery
½ teaspoon (2½ ml) curry powder
¼ teaspoon (2 ml) salt
⅛ teaspoon (1 ml) ground black pepper
2 Tablespoons (30 ml) avocado or olive oil-mayonnaise

Instructions
1. Drain tuna well and place it in a small mixing bowl.
2. Peel, core, and finely chop the apple.
3. Add apple and all remaining ingredients to the bowl with the tuna. Mix well.
4. Sample and adjust salt, pepper, and curry powder to taste.
5. Refrigerate 1 hour if able.

Makes 2 servings
1 serving = 366 calories, 15 g fat, 41 g protein, 13 g carbohydrates, 3 g fiber

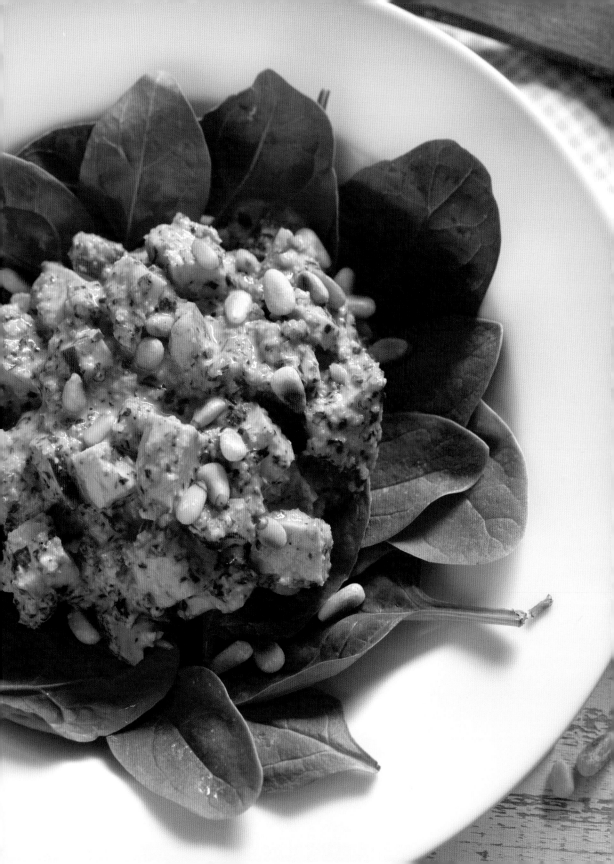

Chopped Pesto Salad

I feel like the food of Europe is pretty universally loved. Maybe that is why I get a look of horror from people when it hits them that they won't be eating regular pasta on an ancestral diet. NO ITALIAN FOOD?! I MIGHT DIE!! No, still Italian food. I agree, we can't go without. I think one of the great things about Europe is that everything is just a bit nicer. The little things. So put this on a pretty dish, add a little garnish, and enjoy it fully.

Prep time: 15 min / Total time: 15 min

Ingredients

4 medium or 2 large vine-ripe tomatoes

6 oz (170 g) cooked chicken

½ cup (120 ml) raw pine nuts

4 cups fresh basil leaves (around 3 oz/85 g with stems still on)

1 clove garlic, peeled

1 teaspoon (5 ml) coconut aminos (optional)

½ teaspoon (2½ ml) sea salt (or to taste)

⅛ teaspoon (½ ml) ground black pepper

¼ cup (60 ml) extra-virgin olive oil

1–3 teaspoons (5–15 ml) water if needed

Salad greens, *or* baby spinach

Instructions

1. Chop tomatoes into large pieces.
2. Cut chicken into 1-inch (2½-cm) pieces.
3. Toast pine nuts in a dry pan on medium heat—watching like a hawk and stirring nearly constantly! It takes only ~1 minute. Stop when nuts are fragrant and/or slightly darkened.
4. In a food processor or blender, combine pine nuts, basil leaves, garlic, coconut aminos, sea salt, pepper, and olive oil until well combined. May add water in 1 teaspoon (5 ml) increments if needed for texture.
5. Toss ¼ cup (60 ml) of this pesto with tomato and chicken. Save leftover pesto for later amazingness.
6. Serve the salad over mixed salad greens or baby spinach. Maybe garnish with a few extra pine nuts.

Makes 3 servings

1 serving = 430 calories, 38 g fat, 19 g protein, 8 g carbohydrates, 2 g fiber

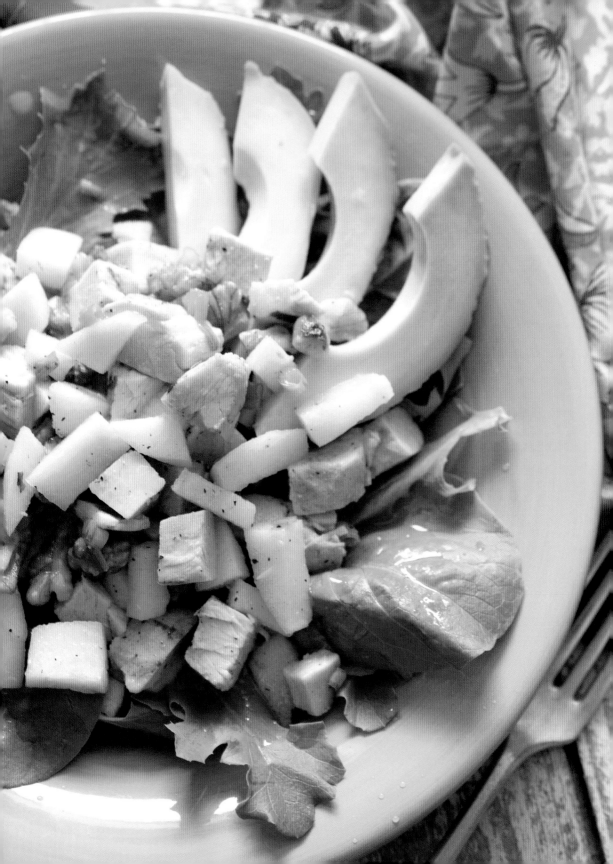

Good Fats Chicken Salad

Fat is back, baby. It turns out we had the whole thing backwards. Eating low-fat everything with refined carbs all the time has resulted in the largest public health crisis of our time: skyrocketing rates of chronic diseases such as obesity, type II diabetes, autoimmune disease, neurodegenerative disease, and cardiovascular disease. You don't need to know all of that to enjoy this salad though. Fat tastes good, especially without the side of guilt.

Prep time: 10 min / Total time: 10 min

Ingredients
3 cups mixed salad greens
3 oz (85 g) cooked chicken (dark meat too!), chopped
1 medium apple, peeled and sliced
½ avocado, cut how you like
2 green onions/scallions, thinly sliced
2 Tablespoons (30 ml) crushed walnuts
1 Tablespoon (15 ml) extra-virgin olive oil
1 teaspoon (5 ml) apple cider vinegar
1 teaspoon (5 ml) honey
Sea salt and ground black pepper to taste

Instructions
1. Place the salad greens in a large bowl and top them with the chicken, apple, avocado, scallions, and walnuts.
2. In a separate bowl, combine olive oil, apple cider vinegar, honey, salt, and pepper. Mix well.
3. Pour half of this dressing over the salad (save leftover dressing for another salad) and enjoy.

Makes 1 serving
1 serving = 531 calories, 32 g fat, 28 g protein, 41 g carbohydrates, 14 g fiber

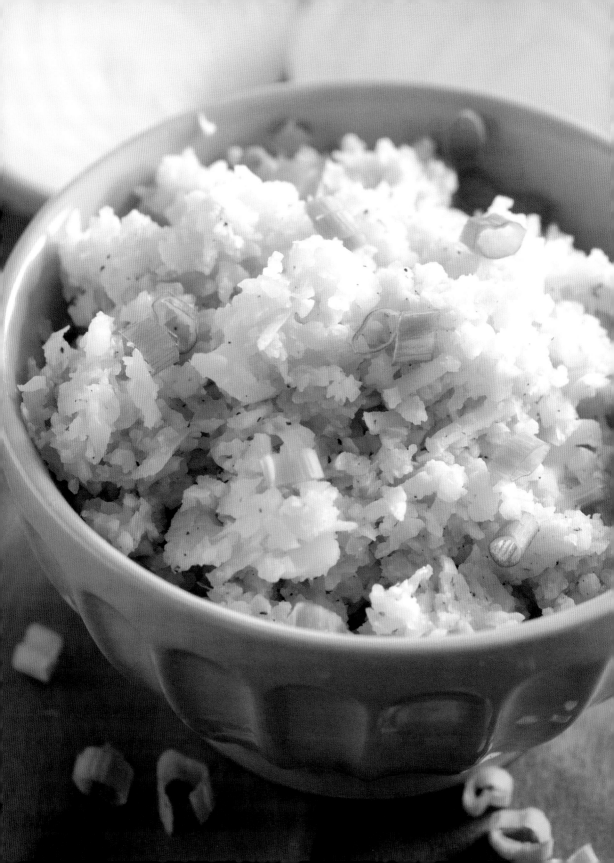

Super Quick Cauliflower Rice

I had a bad experience the first time I tried to make cauliflower rice. I tried to use the low/chopping blade of the food processor. That recipe author is dead to me. Save yourself the agony and use the grating attachment (the big wheel that sits toward the top of the container rather than the bottom). Do the onion and garlic while you're at it. A cheese grater actually works really well also, so either is fine. With a little practice, cauliflower rice will be easy-peasy.

Prep time: 15 min / Total time: 20 min

Ingredients

1 medium head cauliflower
1 yellow onion
2 cloves garlic

1 Tablespoon (15 ml) coconut oil
1 teaspoon (5 ml) sea salt
⅛ teaspoon (1 ml) pepper, or to taste

Instructions

1. Rinse cauliflower under cool water and pat dry. Cut off stem, cut in half, and cut out stem from the two halves.
2. Use a food processor to grate the cauliflower (push it down through grating wheel) and set aside. Grate the onion and set aside. Grate the garlic and set aside. (Alternatively, you can use a cheese grater to grate the cauliflower to a coarse texture, approximately the size of rice grains. Finely chop the onion and garlic.)
3. Heat the coconut oil in a skillet over medium heat.
4. Sauté the onion for 3–4 minutes, or until the onion is relatively translucent. Add the garlic in the final minute.
5. Add in the cauliflower rice and continue to sauté for 4–5 minutes, until softened.
6. Season with salt and pepper and serve.

Makes 4 servings
1 serving = 78 calories, 4 g fat, 3 g protein, 10 g carbohydrates, 4 g fiber

Supercharged Mashed Veg

If you've remained blissfully ignorant of the controversy over white potatoes, then just make this and enjoy it. If you're still scared of them, then feel free to substitute sweet potatoes. Really you only *need* to do this if you have an autoimmune disease or a food sensitivity to white potatoes (solanine in the peel is usually the culprit). Old-school paleo used to exclude them, but really, as long as they're peeled (and this is a meal where you planned to have carbs), you're good.

Prep time: 10 min / Total time: 30 min

Ingredients
2 pounds (1 kg) white potatoes, peeled, *or* sweet potatoes
1 pound (450 g) parsnips, peeled
2 cloves garlic, peeled
2 Tablespoons (30 ml) ghee
~½ cup (120 ml) beef or chicken bone broth
Salt and pepper to taste

Instructions
1. Boil a large pot of water on high heat.
2. Meanwhile, roughly chop peeled potatoes and parsnips. Add vegetables and garlic cloves to your boiling water.
3. Boil vegetables until soft enough to pierce easily with fork.
4. Drain vegetables in colander and return to the empty pot. Add ghee and bone broth to them while still hot and mash well. You may add more broth to reach desired texture, or you may return to heat (stirring frequently) to steam off extra liquid.
5. Season with salt and pepper to taste.

Makes 8 servings
1 serving = 153 calories, 3.7 g fat, 3 g protein, 28 g carbohydrates, 6 g fiber

Roasted Squash Noodles

Love pasta but it doesn't love you back? Try this substitute—it's delicious as a side with a little ghee and salt. You can also serve it with recipes that usually come with pasta, such as stew, goulash, or spaghetti sauce. If you can't find a spaghetti squash, spiralized acorn or butternut squash works. In a pinch, spiralize a zucchini or slice it with a vegetable peeler. Last-ditch effort? Cube a winter squash. You won't get "noodles," but just roast the cubes and use them where you would have had your pasta.

Prep time: 5 min / Cook time: 1 hour / Total time: ~1 hour

Ingredients
1 spaghetti squash (4 lb/2 kg) (Can't find it? See substitute options above.)
1 Tablespoon ghee or coconut oil
Salt and pepper to taste

Instructions
1. Preheat oven to 400°F (200°C).
2. Cut the ends off of your squash, then cut it in half lengthwise. Use a spoon or ice cream scoop to scrape seeds/strings from the center and discard.
3. Place the two squash halves facedown in a large, rimmed roasting pan. Fill the pan with 1" (2½ cm) hot water. Place the pan in your oven.
4. Roast in the oven around 1 hour, rotating the pan at the halfway point. Add a little more water if it completely evaporates. The squash is done when it pierces easily with a fork.
5. Remove the pan from oven and let it cool slightly.
6. Scoop the "noodles" out of the shell/peel and into a bowl. (Careful here! If squash is too hot, it hurts your hand. Trust me on this.)
7. Mix the "noodles" with ghee/oil and salt and pepper to taste.

Makes 6 servings
1 serving = 113 calories, 4 g fat, 2 g protein, 21 g carbohydrates, 5 g fiber

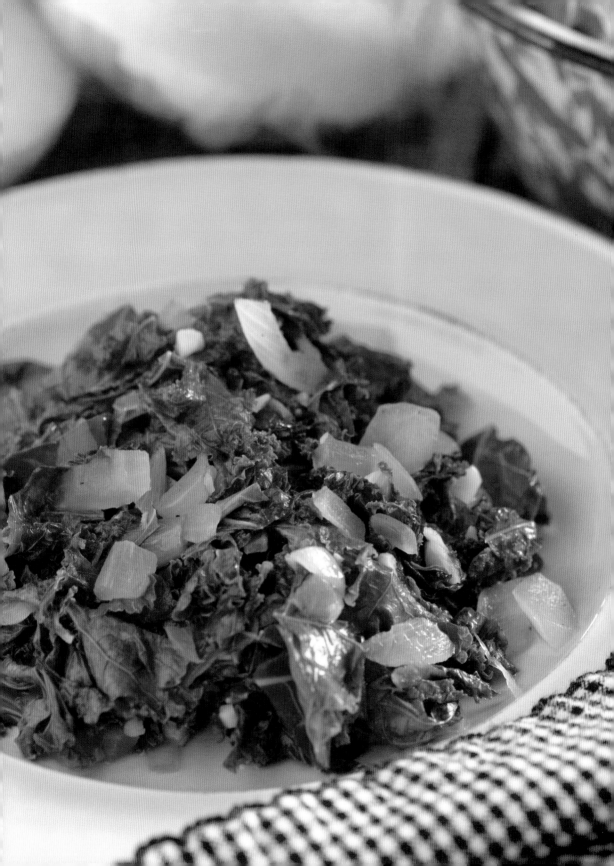

Supercharged Greens

Get on the kale bandwagon, but do it the Southern way. It tastes better this way, I promise. I might not be able to recommend sweet tea or fried dough, but they're getting a lot of things right down there. Like greens.

Prep time: 20 min / Cook time: 30 min / Total time: 30 min

Ingredients

2 Tablespoons (30 ml) fat (skimmed from bone broth), *or* coconut oil

1 medium yellow onion, peeled and chopped

1 large bunch winter greens (collard, chard, or kale)

Salt and pepper to taste

2 garlic cloves, peeled and chopped

½ cup (120 ml) bone broth (any flavor)

Instructions

1. Heat the fat (or coconut oil) in large sauté pan on medium-high heat.
2. Add the chopped onion and sauté until softened.
3. Meanwhile, roughly chop your greens, removing large pieces of stem. Don't worry about the narrower portions of stems toward the upper two-thirds or three-quarters of the leaves. The leaf pieces can be pretty large, up to the size of a playing card (they'll shrink as they cook).
4. Add your chopped greens to the hot pan and season with a little salt and pepper.
5. Cook the greens down for 5–10 minutes, stirring frequently. The heat should be high enough to cook them down but not sear them. You may do this in batches if needed for your pan size.
6. Once the greens are cooked down, add the chopped garlic and sauté until fragrant, about one minute.
7. Add the bone broth and partially cover the pan. Steam the greens, stirring frequently, until stems are fully softened and the broth is mostly cooked down. If needed, add a little water or extra broth if pan gets too dry before greens are fully softened.
8. Feel free to experiment a little! Maybe throw in some nutmeg, anise seeds, cumin . . . whatever sounds good to you. Add any herbs/spices for the final few minutes of cooking.
9. Taste and season to liking with salt and pepper.

Makes 4 servings

1 serving = 107 calories, 7 g fat, 3 g protein, 10 g carbohydrates, 3 g fiber

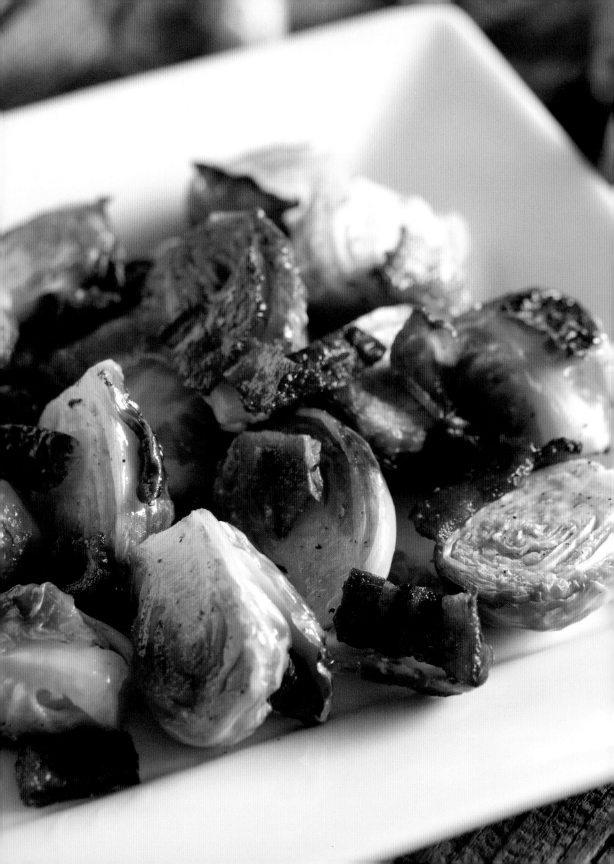

Bacon-Roasted Sprouts

Don't think you like Brussels sprouts? Yeah, I hate them too—when they're plain and steamed. If you haven't tried them roasted with bacon, then you haven't given them a fair chance. These are delicious. In fact, we can take a good lesson from this: bacon is the answer to many food problems.

Prep time: 10 min / Cook time: 40–50 min / Total time: 50–55 min

Ingredients

1½ pounds (680 g) Brussels sprouts
6 pieces bacon (American "streaky" variety)
1 Tablespoon (15 ml) duck fat or coconut oil, melted
¾ teaspoon (4 ml) sea salt (or to taste)
¼ teaspoon (1½ ml) freshly ground black pepper (or to taste)

Instructions

1. Preheat oven to 400°F (200°C).
2. Cut bacon (across) into lardons (thin, ~¼" strips)
3. Cut off the ends of the Brussels sprouts and pull off any yellow outer leaves. Cut each in half (bottom to top).
4. Mix sprouts in a bowl with the oil, salt, and pepper.
5. Pour them on a sheet pan, mix with lardons, and roast for 40–50 minutes, gently tossing every 10 minutes.
6. Remove sprouts from the oven when browned evenly, crisp on the outside, and tender on the inside.
7. Serve immediately.

Makes 6 servings
1 serving = 113 calories, 6 g fat, 7 g protein, 10 g carbohydrates, 4 g fiber

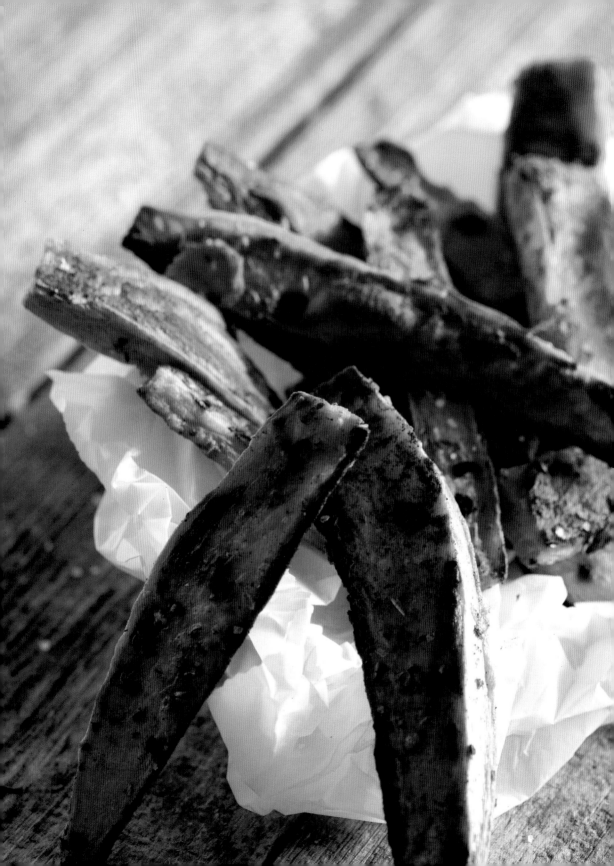

Addicting Sweet Potato Fries

Caution: it's really hard to stop eating these. Make sure you lay them out in a single layer in a hot oven (watch closely) so that they get nice and crispy.

Prep time: 10 min / Cook time: 40 min / Total time: 50 min

Ingredients

3 medium (16 oz/450 g) sweet potatoes, peeled (can leave peel on if desired)
2 Tablespoons (30 ml) melted coconut oil
1 teaspoon (5 ml) pumpkin pie spice (may omit or use cinnamon)
½ teaspoon (2½ ml) dried oregano
¼–½ teaspoon (1–2½ ml) dried hot pepper flakes (spicy! omit if desired)
½ teaspoon sea salt (2½ ml)

Instructions

1. Preheat oven to 425°F (220°C).
2. Cut the potatoes lengthwise into ½" (1 cm) wedges.
3. Toss sweet potato wedges with oil and all spices in a large roasting pan and roast (one layer) in the middle of oven for 10 minutes.
4. Turn wedges over with a spatula and roast them until tender and slightly golden, 20–30 minutes longer (check/turn every 5–10 minutes).

Makes 4 servings
1 serving = 156 calories, 7 g fat, 2 g protein, 23 g carbohydrates, 3 g fiber

Bone Broth Chicken Curry

SO GOOD. It's like takeout but without the tummy ache after. Feel free to sub a curry blend or paste for the individual spices, but just make sure it doesn't have added fillers, preservatives, or coloring. Go as spicy as you like here! I also included a slow cooker version.

Prep time: 30 min / Total time: 70–80 min

Ingredients

1 Tablespoon (15 ml) duck fat, *or* coconut oil, *or* rendered fat from bone broth
1 large onion, chopped
2 Tablespoons (30 ml) finely chopped fresh ginger
4 garlic cloves, chopped
2 pounds/1 kg boneless, skinless chicken thighs, cut into 1–2" pieces
Sea salt and black pepper, to taste
1 Tablespoon (15 ml) curry powder
1 teaspoon (5 ml) turmeric
½ teaspoon (2½ ml) cumin
½ teaspoon (2½ ml) ground coriander
1½ teaspoon (7½ ml) fish sauce (may omit if desired)
1 can (~14 oz or 420 ml) full-fat coconut milk (NOT mixed, just use solids from top—not liquid)
2 cups (480 ml) chicken bone broth
2 cups (480 ml) chopped cabbage
2½ cups carrot slices (~5 medium carrots)
2 cups potato pieces (~5–6 chopped baby potatoes), *or* may sub sweet potato
Super Quick Cauliflower Rice (see page 157), *or* white rice
Unsweetened coconut flakes (optional garnish)

Instructions

1. Melt the fat or coconut oil over medium heat in a large container such as a Dutch oven or big frying pan. (See next page for optional slow cooker version.)
2. Add the onion and ginger. Stir-fry until onion is translucent.
3. Add the garlic and chicken pieces to the pan. Season with salt and pepper.

4. Stir-fry until chicken is nearly fully cooked, then add the curry, turmeric, cumin, and coriander. Stir-fry for ~10 seconds until fragrant.

5. Add the fish sauce, fat from coconut can (may save liquid or discard), chicken bone broth, cabbage, carrots, and potatoes. Adjust heat to simmer while loosely covered (leave slightly askew to allow some steam to escape. Simmer ~30 minutes until veggies are fully cooked, stirring occasionally. Adjust salt and pepper to taste.

6. Serve over choice of Super Quick Cauliflower Rice or white rice (if tolerated). Garnish with a sprinkle of unsweetened coconut flakes. Enjoy!

Makes 8 servings
1 serving (without garnish) = 305 calories, 16 g fat, 26 g protein,
    16 g carbohydrates, 3 g fiber

SLOW COOKER OPTION
Add all ingredients except
1 Tablespoon fat to slow cooker with
veggies on bottom. Cook on low heat
8–10 hours, leaving lid slightly ajar
after 6 hours (to evaporate off extra
liquid). Adjust salt and pepper
to taste.

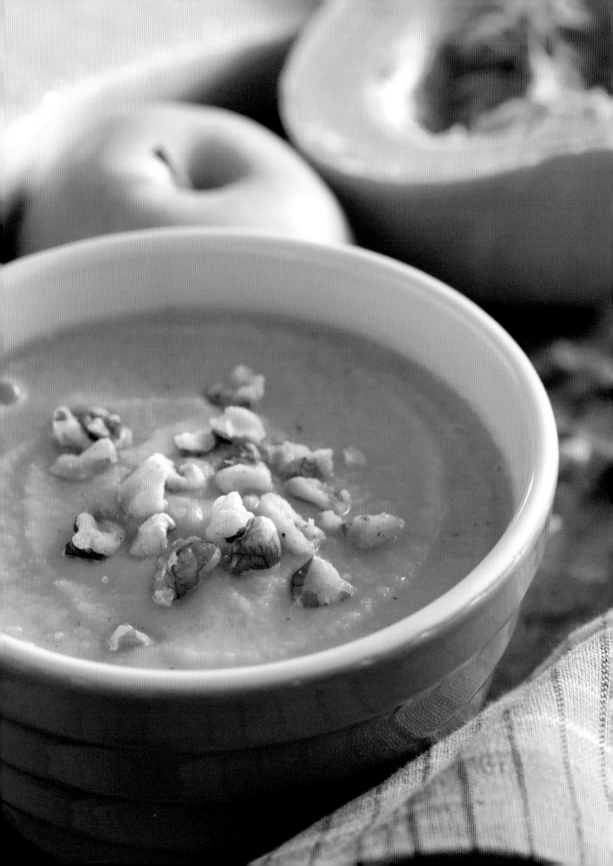

Super Food Soup

Stealth paleo food. This makes a nice, light meal with a salad—but you're still getting a big boost of complete nutrients from the bone broth, veggies, and anti-inflammatory spices. WIN.

Prep time: 30 min / Total time: 30 min

Ingredients

1 butternut squash, *or* ~2 lbs/1 kg pre-peeled and chopped butternut squash cubes
2 Tablespoons (30 ml) coconut oil (or rendered fat from bone broth)
2 medium white or yellow onions (or 1 large), peeled and roughly chopped
3 cloves garlic, peeled and roughly chopped
1 Tablespoon (15 ml) peeled and chopped ginger root
1 medium green apple, peeled, cored, and roughly chopped
4 cups (1 liter) beef bone broth
1 teaspoon (5 ml) turmeric
1 teaspoon (5 ml) nutmeg
Salt and pepper to taste
~4 Tablespoons (60 ml) crushed walnuts (optional garnish)

Instructions

1. If using pre-peeled and chopped squash cubes, go to step 2. If using a whole squash: Cut off stem and base. Cut in half lengthwise. Scoop out and discard seeds. Cut each piece in half the short way, so you'll have quarters. Carefully cut off the peel—the best way is to put the quarter on your cutting board, then hold it down with one palm while sliding the knife down the side. Once peeled, cut each quarter into 1" (2½ cm) cubes.
2. Meanwhile, heat the fat or coconut oil in a large pot or Dutch oven over medium heat and sauté onions until translucent.
3. Add garlic, ginger, apple, and squash cubes. Sauté until the apple softens.
4. Add the broth, turmeric, nutmeg, salt (~½ tsp), and pepper (~⅛ tsp).
5. Cover and simmer until squash is tender (~15 minutes).

Continued on next page.

6. Puree using an immersion blender, blender, or food processor (careful: keep covered well). You may puree in batches. You may add water or additional broth to reach desired texture.
7. Sample and adjust salt and pepper to taste.
8. Garnish with ~1 Tablespoon crushed walnuts per serving.

Makes 4 servings
1 serving = 259 calories, 8 g fat, 8 g protein, 41 g carbohydrates, 7 g fiber

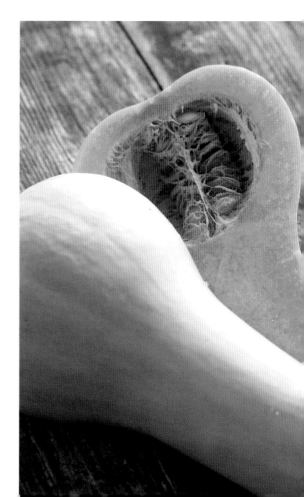

Healing Chicken Soup

I want to eat this *all the time*. You won't miss the noodles, I promise. The bone broth gives it a nice, thick texture. Enjoy it with some extra veggies or a salad on the side, and you've got an easily nourishing, full meal.

Prep time: 20 min / Total time: 90 min

Ingredients

2 Tablespoons (30 ml) coconut oil

2 medium white or yellow onions, peeled and chopped

3 cloves garlic, peeled and finely chopped

1 quart (1 L) Inflammation-Fighting Broth (see recipe on page 120), *or* chicken bone broth

1 head celery, washed and chopped (discard or save both ends for broth)

6 carrots, peeled and chopped (~4 cups)

1 small bunch fresh thyme

1 bay leaf

1 diced jalapeno (optional)

3 pounds (½ kg) cooked, shredded chicken meat (or meat from one roast chicken)

Sea salt and black pepper to taste

Instructions

1. Heat the coconut oil in a large pot or Dutch oven over medium-high heat. Sauté the onions until soft and translucent. Add garlic and sauté until fragrant (1–2 minutes).
2. Add the broth, celery, carrots, thyme, bay leaf, optional jalapeno, and chicken.
3. Bring to a gentle simmer (do not boil).
4. Let simmer approximately 1 hour, stirring occasionally, until vegetables are fully cooked.
5. Season with salt and pepper to taste.

Makes 8 servings

1 serving = 350 calories, 15 g fat, 44 g protein, 8 g carbohydrates, 2 g fiber

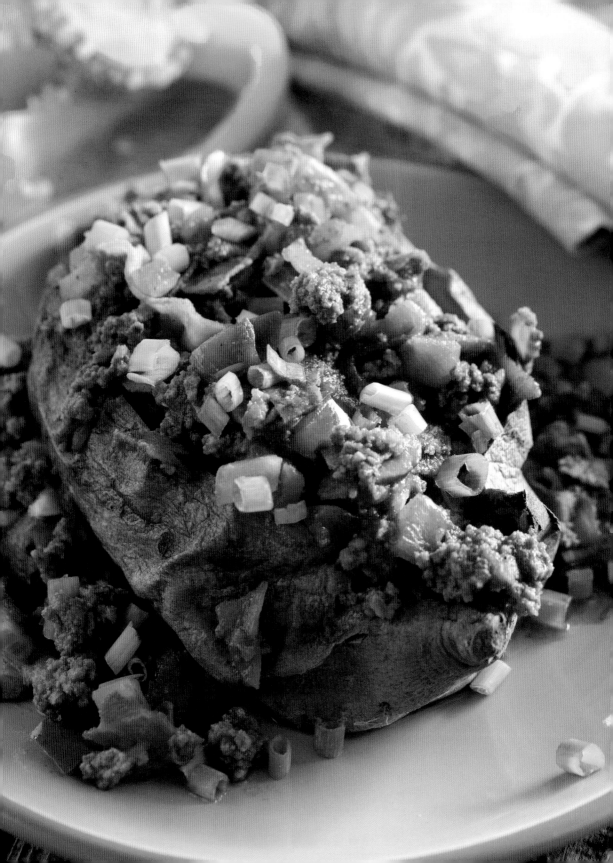

Re-Mix Chili

I know. Chili is another one of those touchy topics. If you're in a group, it's wise not to bring up religion, politics, or your chili recipe. Let's agree on one thing: bacon is delicious. So, call this food whatever you want—chili or "bacon beef food." With tons of clean ingredients, it's going to leave you feeling great.

Prep time: 30 min / Cooking time: 20 min / Total time: 50 min

Ingredients

6 slices American "streaky" bacon

1 white or yellow onion, peeled and diced

2 medium bell peppers (any color), diced

2 cups sliced mushrooms

2 cloves garlic, peeled and minced

1 lb (450 g) grass-fed ground beef

1 teaspoon (5 ml) garlic powder

¼ teaspoon (1 ml) cinnamon

2 teaspoons (10 ml) ground cumin

1 Tablespoon (15 ml) chili powder

1 teaspoon (5 ml) paprika

⅛ teaspoon (1 ml) cayenne pepper (optional, or to taste)

Salt and pepper to taste

1 (14-oz) can crushed tomatoes, undrained

1 (14-oz) can diced tomatoes, drained

1 (4½-oz) small can diced green chilies, drained

1 cup (240 ml) beef broth (bone broth if possible)

Green onions/scallions, sliced (optional garnish)

Instructions

1. Cut the bacon across into lardons (thin, ~¼" strips).
2. Heat the bacon in a large pot or Dutch oven over medium-high heat, stirring frequently, until the fat renders into the pan.
3. Meanwhile, peel and chop the onion, bell peppers, and mushrooms. Add the onion, bell peppers, and mushrooms to your pot. Sauté them with the bacon until the vegetables are softened.
4. Meanwhile, peel and chop the garlic, then add to the pot and sauté 1–2 minutes longer.

Continued on next page.

5. Add the ground beef, garlic powder, cinnamon, cumin, chili powder, paprika, and cayenne pepper. Add salt and pepper if desired. Cook until the beef is browned.
6. Add the crushed and diced tomatoes, green chilies, and broth. Season with salt and pepper.
7. Bring to a simmer and cook, stirring frequently, until cooked down to desired texture (10–20 minutes). Taste and adjust salt and pepper as needed.
8. Serve in a bowl alone, over roasted winter squash, or in a baked sweet potato. Garnish with sliced green onions.

Makes 6 servings
1 serving = 326 calories, 23 g fat, 18 g protein, 14 g carbohydrates, 4 g fiber

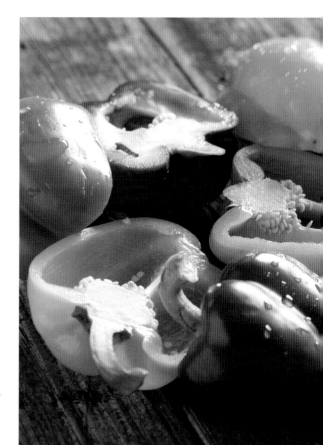

Low-Carb Braised Beef

This cleaned-up braised beef is super filling and comforting. Using all non-starchy vegetables in this recipe gives you the option of having a low-carb meal or of adding something delicious like garlic mashed potatoes on the side. Use bone broth for an extra nutrient boost. The secret to a super-tender roast is low and slow cooking, so make sure you allow plenty of time. This recipe definitely works in a slow cooker (8–10 hours on Low) if you prefer that.

Prep time: 20 min / Total time: ~4 hours

Ingredients
~4 pounds (2 kg) tough beef chuck roast (pot roast)
Salt and pepper to taste
2 Tablespoons (30 ml) beef fat (skimmed from broth) or coconut oil
3 chopped zucchini (courgette)
1 medium white or yellow onion, peeled and
    chopped
3 cups (300 g) chopped celery (4–6 stalks)
3 cups (450 g) stemmed, sliced mushrooms
3 cloves garlic
2 sprigs fresh thyme
2 sprigs fresh rosemary
1½ cups (375 ml) red wine (optional)
1 can (28 oz /~800 ml) chopped tomatoes
2 cups (480 ml) beef bone broth
1 Tablespoon (15 ml) balsamic vinegar

SLOW COOKER OPTION
Add all ingredients to slow cooker in the following order: onions on the bottom, then other veggies/herbs, then meat and liquid. Cook on Low for 8–10 hours.

Instructions
1. Preheat oven to 300°F (150°C).
2. Season roast with salt and pepper to taste.

Continued on next page.

3. Add fat or oil to a large Dutch oven or stock pot, and heat on stove over medium heat.
4. Flick a little water onto fat to test heat. Once pot is hot enough for water to sizzle, sear roast 3–5 minutes per side (until it comes away easily). Set roast aside. (If you're in a huge hurry, you can get away with skipping this step.)
5. In the same hot pot, sauté zucchini, onion, celery, mushrooms, garlic, and salt and pepper to taste until softened (onions are translucent). Add roast, thyme, and rosemary to pot.
6. Add wine (if desired), tomatoes, bone broth, and vinegar. Bring to a gentle simmer.
7. Turn off stove and move pot to oven.
8. Cook with lid cracked for 3–4 hours, until meat pulls apart easily with forks.
9. Taste and season with salt and pepper as desired.
10. Serve with vegetables and juices over meat, or on a side such as mashed root vegetables.

Makes 10 servings
1 serving = 336 calories, 12 g fat, 39 g protein, 10 g carbohydrates, 3 g fiber

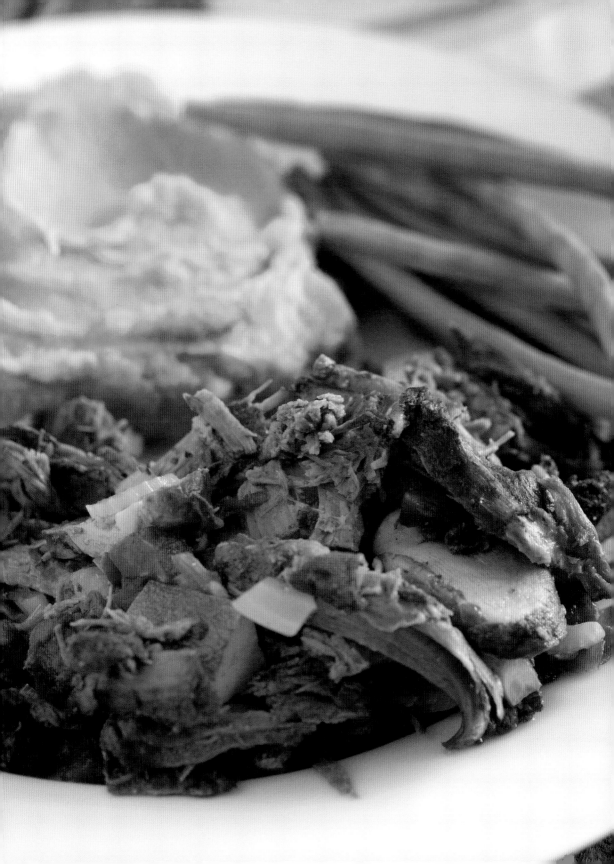

Quickie Roast Chicken

I find that people who roast chickens tend to have strong preferences about their technique. Feel free to roast your chickens however you like. I honestly go all over the place, from slow cooker to very hot oven (like this recipe). The end result is delicious and rewarding: tender chicken and bones to use in your broth. Get there however you like!

Prep time: 20 min / Total time: 2–2½ hours

Ingredients

1 lemon

1 head garlic

1 large white or yellow onion

6 medium carrots

4 parsnips (may sub carrots, sweet potato, or white potato)

1 organic roasting chicken

Salt and pepper to taste

1 bunch fresh thyme

3 Tablespoons (45 ml) ghee or coconut oil, slightly melted (divided)

Kitchen string (optional)

Instructions

1. Preheat your oven to 425°F (220°C).
2. Cut the lemon into quarters, cut the garlic head in half across (cutting all cloves in half), and peel and quarter the onion. Set aside.
3. Peel and roughly chop (into ~2" pieces) the carrots and parsnips. Set aside.
4. Remove and refrigerate any giblets from the chicken.
5. Salt and pepper the inside of the chicken. Stuff it with all of the lemon and garlic and half of the thyme.
6. Place the chicken in a roasting pan and brush or rub all over with 1½ Tablespoons of the melted ghee/oil. Salt and pepper outside of chicken.
7. Position the chicken breast-side-up with wing tips tucked under the body. You may tie the legs together with kitchen string.
8. In a bowl, toss chopped carrots and parsnips, onion, remaining half of thyme, remaining oil/ghee, and salt and pepper to taste.
9. Place these tossed vegetables around the chicken in the roasting pan (or in a separate pan if preferred).

10. Roast the chicken for about 70–90 minutes, or until juices run clear in hip joint (cut between thigh and body to check juice). The internal temperature in this joint should reach 160°F (70°C).
11. Let the chicken rest, covered, for 10–15 minutes before cutting.

Makes 6 servings
1 serving = 297 calories, 11 g fat, 26 g protein, 26 g carbohydrates, 6 g fiber

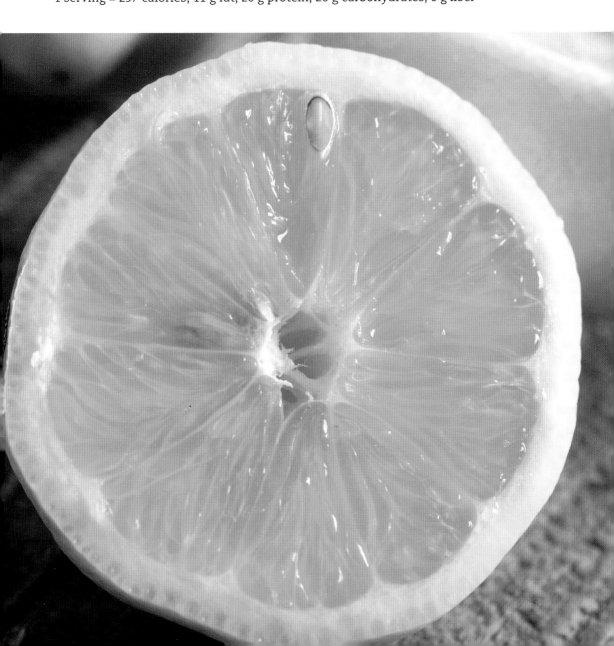

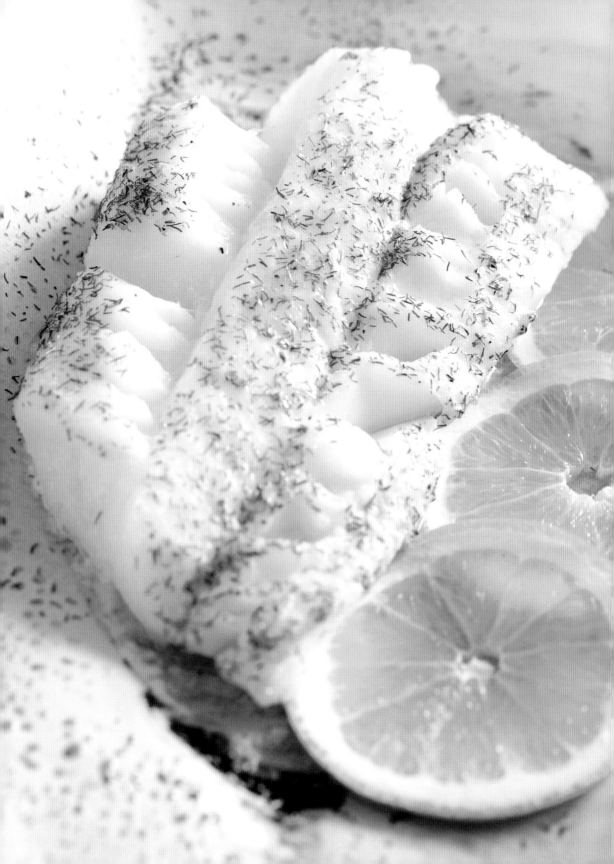

Sunny Day Fish

Whether it's a sunny day or not, this fish will bring some sparkle to your day. As a California native, this meal brings me home no matter where in the world I am. If you don't have access to sea bass, feel free to substitute a different firm white fish.

Prep time: 10 min / Total time: 20 min

Ingredients
1 medium orange (will need zest from half and 2 Tablespoons/30 ml juice)
1 Tablespoon (15 ml) raw, local honey
1 Tablespoon (15 ml) Dijon mustard
2 teaspoons (10 ml) extra-virgin olive oil, divided
¼ teaspoon sea salt
⅛ teaspoon black pepper
1 lb (450 g) sea bass fillets (or other firm white fish such as tilapia, halibut, pollock, mahi mahi, cod, or sole)
Several sprigs fresh dill (or may substitute dried dill)

Instructions
1. Preheat oven to 400°F (200°C).
2. Mix zest of half the orange, 2 Tablespoons orange juice, honey, mustard, 1 teaspoon olive oil, ¼ teaspoon salt, and ⅛ teaspoon black pepper in a small bowl. Brush or drizzle this mixture onto both sides of the fish fillets.
3. Coat the bottom of a glass or ceramic baking dish with 1 teaspoon olive oil.
4. Place fish in baking dish, skin-side down (if it has skin). Place 1–2 sprigs of dill on top of each fillet (or sprinkle fish with dried dill).
5. Place the pan in the oven and bake it about 10 minutes, until fish is cooked throughout and flakes easily in the middle.

Makes 3 servings
1 serving = 231 calories, 9 g fat, 29 g protein, 8 g carbohydrates, 0 g fiber

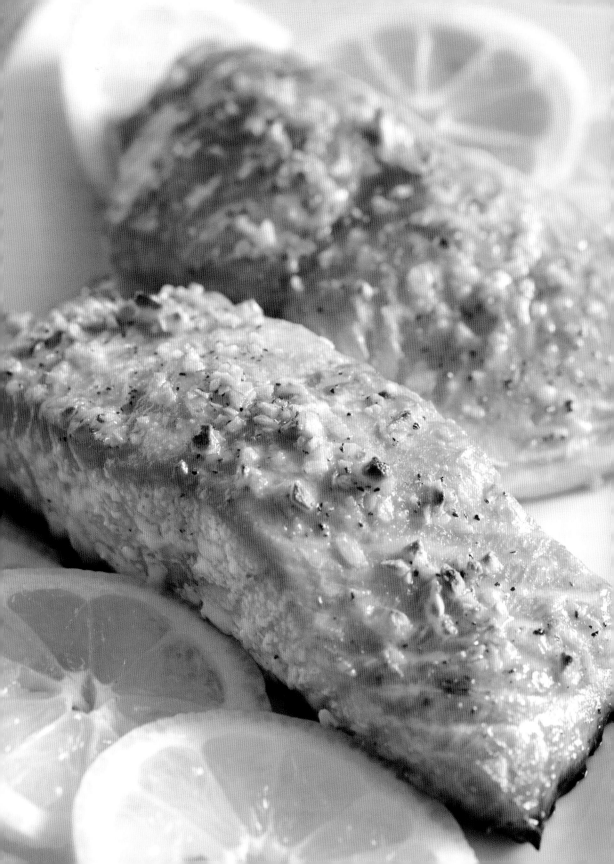

Maple Roast Salmon

So simple. So good. This recipe calls for coconut aminos, an ancestral substitute for soy sauce. Check online and at health food stores to find it. In a pinch, you can omit it or substitute gluten-free fish sauce for a little umami.

Prep time: 10 min / Cook time: 20 min / Total time: 1 hour

Ingredients
¼ cup (60 ml) pure maple syrup
2 Tablespoons (30 ml) coconut aminos
2 cloves garlic, minced
½ teaspoon (1½ ml) sea salt, or to taste
⅛ teaspoon (1 ml) ground black pepper, or to taste
1 lb (450 g) fresh salmon
Lemon slices or fresh herbs (optional garnish)

Instructions
1. To make the marinade: combine maple syrup, coconut aminos, garlic, salt, and pepper in a bowl.
2. Place fish in a shallow baking dish. Top with marinade, coating both sides. Cover the dish.
3. Refrigerate your fish for 30 minutes, turning once.
4. Meanwhile, preheat your oven to 400°F (200°C).
5. Ensure that fish are skin-side down in dish. Place the dish in the oven uncovered for 15–20 minutes. The fish is done when it flakes easily with a fork.
6. Serve garnished with lemon slices or chopped fresh herbs.

Makes 3 servings
1 serving = 290 calories, 10 g fat, 31 g protein, 18 g carbohydrates, 1 g fiber

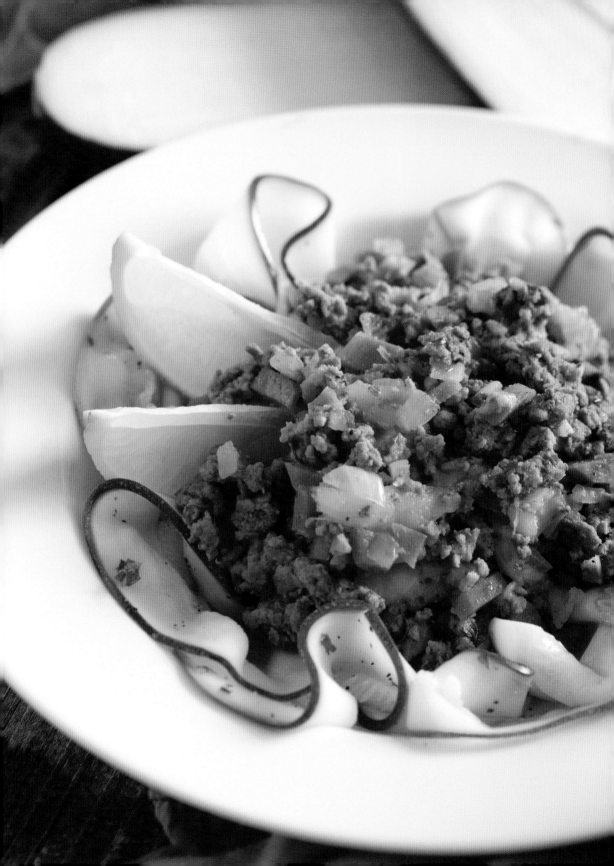

Baba Ganoush Lamb with Zucchini Noodles

The Middle East. The Mediterranean. The UK. What do they all have in common? Lamb is everywhere—and it's amazing. No matter where you live, you can go on a little vacation with this meal. If you don't have the good fortune of having access to lamb, you can substitute ground beef.

Prep time: 30 min / Total time: 40 min

Ingredients

2 medium (or 1 large) eggplant (aubergine)
2 Tablespoons (30 ml) coconut oil, melted
Salt and pepper to taste
1 medium white or yellow onion
1 medium carrot
1 lb (450 g) ground lamb (mince), or sub ground beef
½ cup (120 ml) bone broth (ideally beef or lamb)
¼ cup (60 ml) chermoula paste (from jar or make your own on page 187)
2 medium zucchini (courgette)
1 Tablespoon (15 ml) extra-virgin olive oil
3 Tablespoons (45 ml) fresh mint, chopped
1 lime

NOTE

If you're making your own chermoula paste, whip up a batch before diving into step 2 (see recipe on page 187). You will use ¼ cup in this recipe and refrigerate or freeze the rest for later use.

Instructions

1. Preheat oven to 430°F (220°C).
2. Cut the eggplant in half lengthwise. Make deep cuts (through the flesh but not the peel) diagonally in a crisscross pattern, spaced about ½" apart.
3. Rub each eggplant half all over with melted coconut oil (save remaining oil). Sprinkle the tops with salt and pepper.
4. Put your eggplant halves on a roasting pan in the oven for 20–30 minutes (until soft throughout).

Continued on next page.

5. Meanwhile, peel and finely chop the onion. Peel the carrot and dice it.
6. Heat remaining coconut oil in a pan on medium heat. Add the carrot and onion and sauté until softened, around 5 minutes.
7. Add the lamb and season with ¼ teaspoon salt and a little bit of pepper. Break up/stir until no longer pink.
8. Drain extra fat from the pan.
9. Add bone broth and chermoula paste. Cook about 5 minutes, until moisture is cooked down.
10. Once eggplants are done (soft throughout and browned), remove them from the oven and let cool. Use a spoon or your hands to scoop the eggplant flesh out of the skin, and add it to the lamb mixture (discard skin).
11. Mix lamb/eggplant mixture, gently heat, and taste. Adjust seasoning as desired.
12. Meanwhile, use a vegetable peeler to peel the zucchini into flat strips (discard ends). You may stop when you get to the seed part. (Alternately, you may use a spiralizer.)
13. Steam your zucchini "noodles" very briefly, only 2–3 minutes. Combine zucchini "noodles" with the olive oil, chopped mint, salt, and pepper.
14. Cut lime into wedges and serve with the lamb mixture and zucchini noodles.

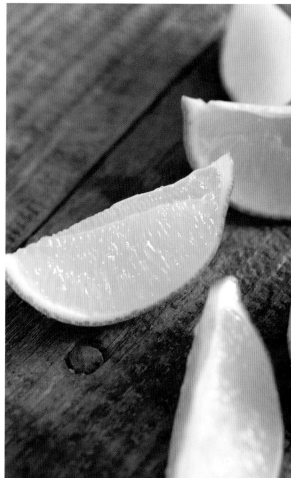

Makes 5 servings
1 serving = 399 calories, 30 g fat, 18 g protein, 16 g carbohydrates, 8 g fiber

Chermoula Paste

If only we could all jet off to Morocco for an amazing food-cation. If that's not in the cards, then you don't have to settle for jarred chermoula paste. There are endless variations on this marinade/sauce for meat and/or fish. Pickled or preserved lemons are a great substitution for the lemon juice. You can add/ substitute any hot peppers you like for the cayenne.

Prep time: 5 min / Total time: 5 min

Ingredients
1 cup (240 ml) packed fresh cilantro/coriander
¼ cup (60 ml) packed fresh parsley
2 peeled garlic cloves
2 Tablespoons (30 ml) lemon juice
½ Tablespoon (7½ ml) paprika
1 teaspoon (5 ml) ground cumin
¼ teaspoon (1 ml) cayenne pepper
¼ cup (60 ml) extra-virgin olive oil
½ teaspoon (2½ ml) sea salt, or to taste

Instructions
1. Combine cilantro, parsley, garlic, lemon juice, paprika, cumin, cayenne, olive oil, and salt in a food processor or blender.
2. Use this paste as a marinade or sauce for fish or meat.
3. You may refrigerate/freeze the leftovers for later use.

Makes 10 servings
1 serving = 50 calories, 5.4 g fat, 0.1 g protein, 0.6 g carbohydrates, 0.1 g fiber

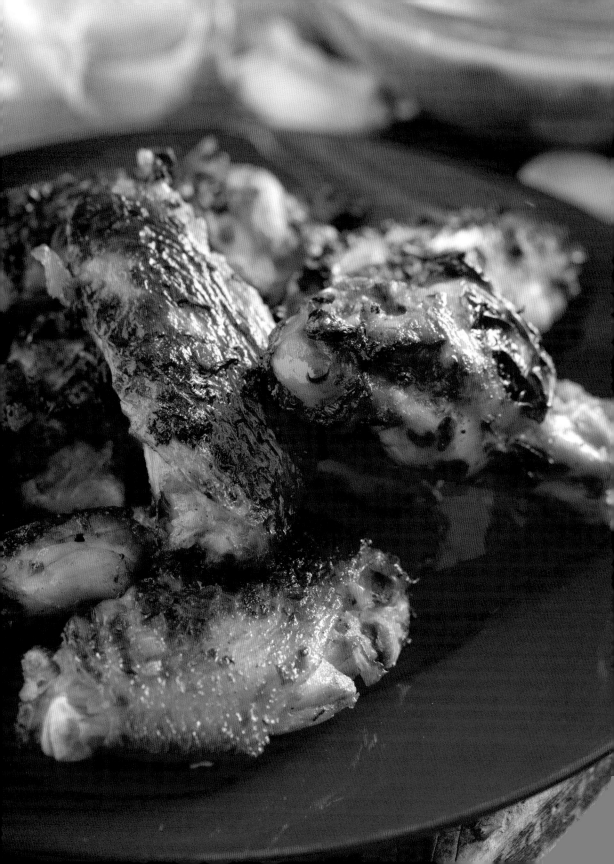

Sweet & Spicy Wings

You might not think these ingredients go together, but just listen to the crazy bone broth lady: it's delicious. DON'T THROW AWAY THOSE BONES. Because broth.

Prep time: 30 min / Cook time: 30 min / Marinate time: 4–12 hours / Total time: 5–13 hours

Ingredients

1 14-oz (400-ml) can crushed tomatoes
½ medium onion, peeled and *finely* chopped
2 large pieces of jarred, roasted red peppers, chopped
2 jarred green chilies, very finely chopped (optional, or to taste)
⅓ cup apple cider vinegar
1 teaspoon (5 ml) sea salt

¼ teaspoon (1 ml) ground cloves
1 stick cinnamon or ¼ teaspoon (1 ml) ground cinnamon
⅓ cup (80 ml) pure maple syrup
½ cup (120 ml) bone broth
2 Tablespoons (30 ml) Dijon mustard
2 pounds (1 kg) bone-in chicken wings (best quality you can find)

Instructions

1. In a medium pot, combine crushed tomatoes, onion, roasted peppers, green chilis, apple cider vinegar, sea salt, cloves, cinnamon, maple syrup, and bone broth. Bring to a simmer.
2. Turn heat down to medium-low and simmer for about 10 minutes, stirring and breaking up tomato pieces, until slightly reduced. Turn off heat.
3. Add Dijon mustard and stir to combine.
4. Let cool in refrigerator if possible, or at least cool slightly in freezer for a few minutes.
5. Add chicken wings and stir to coat. Marinate for 4–12 hours.
6. Preheat broiler to medium. (Alternatively, preheat oven to 375°F/190°C. Or you may use a grill.)

Continued on next page.

7. Remove chicken from marinade, letting the excess fall off, and saving the extra marinade. Place the chicken on a foil-lined oven or grill pan.
8. Cook chicken wings 4" from broiler for 12–20 minutes, basting with extra marinade and turning every few minutes. (Alternatively, you may bake them in the oven for 30–40 minutes, basting and turning every 10–15 minutes.) *Do not add marinade during the final five minutes.*
9. Wings are done when juices run clear and/or internal temperature reaches 165°F (75°C).

Makes 4 servings
1 serving = 379 calories, 8 g fat, 49 g protein, 27 g carbohydrates, 3 g fiber

Cleaned-Up Ranch

That bottle of ranch dressing lurking in your fridge . . . it's hiding some dirty little secrets on the ingredient list. Introducing: the solution. You might need a trivia game, some crudités, and some chicken wings to go with this.

Prep time: 10 min / Total time: 10 min + 2 hours to chill if possible

Ingredients
½ cup (120 ml) chilled coconut milk from can (mix *well* before measuring)
1 clove garlic, crushed or finely grated
½ teaspoon (2½ ml) onion powder
1 Tablespoon (15 ml) chopped fresh dill
½ teaspoon (2½ ml) white vinegar
¼ teaspoon (1 ml) paprika
~⅛ teaspoon (½ ml) or to taste cayenne or black pepper
¼ teaspoon (1 ml) sea salt
½ cup (120 ml) chilled clean mayonnaise (store-bought, made with avocado or
   olive oil, *or* make your own)

Instructions
1. Empty coconut milk can into a bowl and combine well (until consistent texture/
   no lumps).
2. In a bowl, combine ½ cup of the coconut milk, garlic, onion powder, dill,
   vinegar, paprika, cayenne, salt, and mayonnaise and mix well.
3. Chill your mixture in the refrigerator ~2 hours if possible.

Makes 8 servings (1 serving = 2 Tablespoons)
1 serving = 63 calories, 7 g fat, 0 g protein, 1 g carbohydrates, 0 g fiber

Resources

My genuine wish is for you to be successful during the twenty-one-day program and beyond. So here are some of my personal favorite places to find recipes, ingredients, and information. I have no affiliation with any of the resources listed except for, of course, my own website and the healthcare professional directories where I am listed.

Recipes

If you need to add more recipes, no problem. Make sure that when you add a new recipe to the plan, you still follow the template from Chapter 9. Avoid trying to re-create paleo versions of baked goods (i.e. "paleo cookies"), especially if you're working on weight loss. There are a ton of free paleo recipes and websites, so feel free to browse around. Here are a few that I frequent:

- Balanced Bites/Practical Paleo: http://balancedbites.com/recipes/
- Nom Nom Paleo: http://nomnompaleo.net/recipeindex/
- PaleOMG: http://paleomg.com/
- Against All Grain: http://againstallgrain.com/
- Autoimmune Paleo: http://autoimmune-paleo.com
- Well Fed: http://meljoulwan.com/category/recipes/
- Sarah Fragoso: http://sarahfragoso.com/recipes/
- Paleo Comfort Foods: http://paleocomfortfoods.com/category/recipes/
- Paleo Parents (good for kids): http://paleoparents.com/tag/recipe/
- Nourished Kitchen (recipes for fermented foods): http://nourishedkitchen.com/recipe-index/ferments-cultured-food/

Ingredients and Products

Need sources for quality paleo ingredients? Here are some online options:

- Thrive Market—kind of like an online Costco for natural foods (US only): https://thrivemarket.com
- Amazon—lots of paleo foods that can be hard to find in stores: www.amazon.com

- Tropical Traditions—everything coconut and much more: http://tropicaltraditions.com/
- US Wellness Meats—an online source for grass-fed and organic bones (ships within US): http://grasslandbeef.com
- The Brothery—purchase bone broth online within the US: https://www.bonebroth.com
- The Paleo Broth Company—purchase bone broth online within the UK (ships anywhere within UK except the Highlands): http://www.thepaleobrothcompany.com/

Also look into local ways to procure quality foods. Look for a Community Supported Agriculture (CSA) produce box program; they provide boxes of local, organic produce by subscription. Also look for meat/egg co-ops. These often allow you to either purchase a large box of grass-fed beef and/or go in with some friends to purchase a portion of a grass-fed animal. Sometimes poultry, eggs, etc. are also offered. The USDA database is a good place to start: https://www.ams.usda.gov/local-food-directories/csas

The Environmental Working Group (EWG) provides two important resources:

- The Dirty Dozen and Clean 15 lists of produce with the most and least pesticide residue: https://www.ewg.org/foodnews
- The Skin Deep Cosmetics Database grades the safety of personal care products: http://www.ewg.org/skindeep/

Learn More

Here are some good places to learn more about bone broth, ancestral diets, and functional medicine/nutrition:

- Weston A. Price Foundation: http://www.westonaprice.org
- Chris Kresser: http://chriskresser.com/
- Chris Masterjohn, PhD—The Daily Lipid Podcast: http://chrismasterjohnphd.com/podcast/
- Robb Wolf: http://robbwolf.com/
- Dr. Ruscio: http://drruscio.com/
- Ancestral RDs Podcast: http://theancestralrds.com/

- Health Edge Podcast: http://www.thehealthedgepodcast.com/
- Mark's Daily Apple: http://www.marksdailyapple.com/

Get Help

Although bone broth and an ancestral approach to nutrition are a great way to start, it sometimes takes more. If you aren't able to experience the full results that you desire from the guidance in this book, then I recommend working with a professional. If your goals are health-related, then always start with your physician. However, even many physicians will admit that the conventional healthcare approach is better equipped for acute illness and injury than it is for treatment of chronic disease. There is a growing number of functional and ancestral medicine practitioners who aim to address root causes and to treat without pharmacological intervention whenever possible. Below are some ways to learn more and to find such a practitioner:

- Real Nutrition RX—This is my private practice. I work virtually with clients in the United States and the United Kingdom: www.RealNutritionRX.com
- Academy of Nutrition and Dietetics "Find an Expert"—Make sure you filter for the expertise area of "Integrative & Functional Nutrition": http://www.eatright.org/find-an-expert
- Dietitians in Integrative and Functional Medicine: http://integrativerd.org
- Primal Docs "Find a Practitioner": http://primaldocs.com/members/
- The Institute for Functional Medicine: https://www.functionalmedicine.org

References

Chapter 1. An Ancient Food

Bengmark, Stig. "Obesity, the Deadly Quartet and the Contribution of the Neglected Daily Organ Rest—A New Dimension of Un-Health and Its Prevention." *Hepatobiliary Surgery and Nutrition* 4, no. 4 (August 4, 2015): 278–88. doi:10.3978/j.issn.2304-3881.2015.07.02.

Boyle, Coleen A., Sheree Boulet, Laura A. Schieve, Robin A. Cohen, Stephen J. Blumberg, Marshalyn Yeargin-Allsopp, Susanna Visser, et al. "Trends in the Prevalence of Developmental Disabilities in US Children, 1997–2008." *Pediatrics* 127, no. 6 (June 2011): 1034–42. doi: 10.1542/peds.2010-2989

CDC. "Attention Deficit Hyperactive Disorder." May 4, 2016. Accessed June 8, 2016. http://www.cdc.gov/ncbddd/adhd/data.html.

CDC. "Autism Spectrum Disorder." March 31, 2016. Accessed June 8, 2016. http://www.cdc.gov/ncbddd/autism/data.html.

CDC. "Changes in Life Expectancy by Race and Hispanic Origin in the United States, 2013–2014." April 20, 2016. Accessed June 13, 2016. http://www.cdc.gov/nchs/products/databriefs/db244.htm.

CDC. "Leading Causes of Death." April 27, 2016. Accessed June 13, 2016. http://www.cdc.gov/nchs/fastats/leading-causes-of-death.htm.

CDC. "Osteoporosis." September 29, 2015. Accessed June 8, 2016. http://www.cdc.gov/nchs/fastats/osteoporosis.htm.

Cohn, D'Vera. "The Growing Global Chronic Disease Epidemic." *Population Reference Bureau.* May 2007. http://www.prb.org/Publications/Articles/2007/GrowingGlobalChronicDiseaseEpidemic.aspx.

Fulgoni, Victor L., Debra R. Keast, Regan L. Bailey, and Johanna Dwyer. "Foods, Fortificants, and Supplements: Where Do Americans Get Their Nutrients?" *The Journal of Nutrition* 141, no. 10 (October 1, 2011): 1847–54. doi:10.3945/jn.111.142257.

Gao, J., J. Wu, X. N. Zhao, W. N. Zhang, Y. Y. Zhang, and Z. X. Zhang. "Transplacental Neurotoxic Effects of Monosodium Glutamate on Structures and Functions of Specific Brain Areas of Filial Mice." *Sheng Li Xue Bao* 46, no. 1 (February 1994): 44–51.

Gibbons, Gary H. "What Are the Health Risks of Overweight and Obesity?" November 12, 2013. Accessed June 13, 2016. https://www.nhlbi.nih.gov/health/health-topics/topics/obe/risks.

Meetoo, Danny. "Chronic Diseases: The Silent Global Epidemic." *British Journal of Nursing* 17, no. 21 (November 2008): 1320–25. doi:10.12968/bjon.2008.17.21.31731.

Morell, Sally Fallon, and Kaayla T. Daniel. *Nourishing Broth: An Old-Fashioned Remedy for the Modern World.* New York: Grand Central Life & Style, 2014.

National Institutes of Health—The Autoimmune Diseases Coordinating Committee. *Progress in Autoimmune Diseases Research.* n.p.: U.S. Department of Health and Human Services, 2005. https://www.niaid.nih.gov/topics/autoimmune/Documents/adccfinal.pdf.

Ng, Marie, Tom Fleming, Margaret Robinson, Blake Thomson, Nicholas Graetz, Christopher Margono, Erin C. Mullany, et al. "Global, Regional, and National Prevalence of Overweight and Obesity in Children and Adults During 1980–2013: A Systematic Analysis for the Global Burden of Disease Study 2013." *The Lancet* 384, no. 9945 (August 30, 2014): 766–81. doi:10.1016/S0140-6736(14)60460-8.

Office of the Assistant Secretary for Planning and Evaluation. "Action Against Asthma: A Strategic Plan for the Department of Health and Human Services. Epidemic of a Chronic Disease." *U.S. Department of Health & Human Services*. May 1, 2001. Accessed June 8, 2016. https://aspe.hhs.gov/report/action-against-asthma-strategic-plan-department-health-and-human-services/epidemic-chronic-disease

Poti, Jennifer M., Michelle A. Mendez, Shu Wen Ng, and Barry M. Popkin. "Is the Degree of Food Processing and Convenience Linked with the Nutritional Quality of Foods Purchased by US Households?" *The American Journal of Clinical Nutrition* 101, no. 6 (June 2015): 1251–62. doi:10.3945/ajcn.114.100925.

Quann, Erin E., Victor L. Fulgoni, and Nancy Auestad. "Consuming the Daily Recommended Amounts of Dairy Products Would Reduce the Prevalence of Inadequate Micronutrient Intakes in the United States: Diet Modeling Study Based on NHANES 2007–2010." *Nutrition Journal* 14, no. 90 (September 4, 2015). doi:10.1186/s12937-015-0057-5.

Rennard, Barbara O., Ronald F. Ertl, Gail L. Gossman, Richard A. Robbins, and Stephen I. Rennard. "Chicken Soup Inhibits Neutrophil Chemotaxis in Vitro." *Chest* 118, no. 4 (October 2000): 1150–57. doi:10.1378/chest.118.4.1150.

Scollon, Christie Napa, and Ed Diener. "Love, Work, and Changes in Extraversion and Neuroticism over Time." *Journal of Personality and Social Psychology* 91, no. 6 (December 2006): 1152–65. doi.org/10.1037/0022-3514.91.6.1152.

Spreadbury, Ian. "Comparison with Ancestral Diets Suggests Dense Acellular Carbohydrates Promote an Inflammatory Microbiota, and May Be the Primary Dietary Cause of Leptin Resistance and Obesity." *Diabetes, Metabolic Syndrome and Obesity: Targets and Therapy* 2012, no. 5 (July 2012): 175–89. doi:10.2147/dmso.s33473.

Twenge, Jean M., Brittany Gentile, C. Nathan DeWall, Debbie Ma, Katharine Lacefield, and David R. Schurtz. "Birth Cohort Increases in Psychopathology Among Young Americans, 1938–2007: A Cross-Temporal Meta-Analysis of the MMPI." *Clinical Psychology Review* 30, no. 2 (March 2010): 145–54. doi:10.1016/j.cpr.2009.10.005.

U.S. Food and Drug Administration. "Questions and Answers on Monosodium Glutamate (MSG)." July 22, 2014. Accessed June 8, 2016. http://www.fda.gov/Food/IngredientsPackagingLabeling/FoodAdditivesIngredients/ucm328728.htm

Wu, Renee. "Is MSG Bad for You?" *Yale Scientific Magazine*. April 3, 2011. http://www.yalescientific.org/2011/04/is-msg-bad-for-you/

Chapter 2. Beneficial Components
&
Chapter 3. Bone Broth Healing Powers

Aalto, Maija, Kirsti Lampiaho, J. Pikkarainen, and E. Kulonen. "Amino Acid Metabolism of Experimental Granulation Tissue in Vitro." *Biochemical Journal* 132, no. 4 (April 1973): 663–71. doi:10.1042/bj1320663.

Abraham, William, and Monsanto Technology LLC. Glyphosate formulations and their use for the inhibition of 5-enolpyruvylshikimate-3-phosphate synthase. US Patent 7771736 B2, filed August 29, 2003, and issued August 10, 2010.

Airaksinen, K. E. J., P. I. Salmela, M. K. Linnaluoto, M. J. Ikaheimo, K. Ahola, and L. J. Ryhanen. "Diminished Arterial Elasticity in Diabetes: Association with Fluorescent Advanced Glycosylation End Products in Collagen." *Cardiovascular Research* 27, no. 6 (June 1, 1993): 942–45. doi:10.1093/cvr/27.6.942.

"Alanine: Amino Acid Health Benefits, Dietary Sources, Side Effects." *Vitamins & Health Supplements Guide.* 2005. Accessed May 31, 2016. http://www.vitamins-supplements.org/amino-acids/alanine.php

Albina, Jorge E., Joseph A. Abate, and Balduino Mastrofrancesco. "Role of Ornithine as a Proline Precursor in Healing Wounds." *Journal of Surgical Research* 55, no. 1 (July 1993): 97–102. doi:10.1006/jsre.1993.1114.

Albrecht, Jan. "Glutamine in the Central Nervous System: Function and Dysfunction." *Frontiers in Bioscience* 12, no. 1 (2007): 332–43. doi:10.2741/2067.

Allen, John, and John F. Prudden. "Histologic Response to a Cartilage Powder Preparation in a Controlled Human Study." *The American Journal of Surgery* 112, no. 6 (December 1966): 888–91. doi:10.1016/0002-9610(66)90144-9.

American Society of Nephrology. "Calcium Supplements May Increase the Risk of Kidney Stone Recurrence." *Science Daily.* October 13, 2015. https://www.sciencedaily.com/releases/2015/10/151013103619.htm

Amores-Sánchez, María Isabel, and Miguel Ángel Medina. "Glutamine, as a Precursor of Glutathione, and Oxidative Stress." *Molecular Genetics and Metabolism* 67, no. 2 (June 1999): 100–105. doi:10.1006/mgme.1999.2857.

Berlett, B. S., and E. R. Stadtman. "Protein Oxidation in Aging, Disease, and Oxidative Stress." *Journal of Biological Chemistry* 272, no. 33 (August 15, 1997): 20313–16. doi:10.1074/jbc.272.33.20313.

Bittigau, P., and C. Ikonomidou. "Topical Review: Glutamate in Neurologic Diseases." *Journal of Child Neurology* 12, no. 8 (November 1, 1997): 471–85. doi:10.1177/088307389701200802.

Bolland, M. J., A. Avenell, J. A. Baron, A. Grey, G. S. MacLennan, G. D. Gamble, and I. R. Reid. "Effect of Calcium Supplements on Risk of Myocardial Infarction and Cardiovascular Events: Meta-Analysis." *The BMJ* 341, no. c3691 (July 2010). doi:10.1136/bmj.c3691.

Bolland, Mark J., William Leung, Vicky Tai, Sonja Bastin, Greg D Gamble, Andrew Grey, and Ian R Reid. "Calcium Intake and Risk of Fracture: Systematic Review." *The BMJ* 351, no. h4580 (September 29, 2015). doi:10.1136/bmj.h4580.

Brind, Joel, Virginia Malloy, Nicholas Caliendo, Joseph Vogelman, Jay Zimmerman, and Norman Orentreich. "Dietary Glycine Supplementation Mimics Lifespan Extension by Dietary Methionine Restriction in Fisher 344 Rats." *The FASEB Journal* 25, no. 1 (April 2011). http://www.fasebj.org/content/25/1_Supplement/528.2?related-urls=yes&legid=fasebj;25/1_Supplement/528.2

Brooks, Susan, Anthony Leathem, and Miriam Dwek. "Altered Expression of N-Acetyl Galactosamine Glycoproteins by Breast Cancers." *Biochemical Society Transactions* 22, no. 2 (May 1994): 95S. doi:10.1042/bst022095s.

Bruyere, Olivier, and Jean-Yves Reginster. "Glucosamine and Chondroitin Sulfate as Therapeutic Agents for Knee and Hip Osteoarthritis." *Drugs & Aging* 24, no. 7 (July 2007): 573–80. doi:10.2165/00002512-200724070-00005.

Calder, P. C. "Glutamine and the Immune System." *Clinical Nutrition* 13, no. 1 (February 1994): 2–8. doi:10.1016/0261-5614(94)90003-5.

Campbell-McBride, Natasha. "About." Accessed June 30, 2016. http://www.gapsdiet.com/about.html

Castelo-Branco, C., M. Duran, and J. González-Merlo. "Skin Collagen Changes Related to Age and Hormone Replacement Therapy." *Maturitas* 15, no. 2 (October 1992): 113–19. doi:10.1016/0378-5122(92)90245-y.

Cervigni, Mauro. "Interstitial Cystitis/Bladder Pain Syndrome and Glycosaminoglycans Replacement Therapy." *Translational Andrology and Urology* 4, no. 6 (December 7, 2015): 638–42. doi:10.3978/j.issn.2223-4683.2015.11.04.

Chen, Jeen-Kuan, Chia-Rui Shen, and Chao-Lin Liu. "N-Acetylglucosamine: Production and Applications." *Marine Drugs* 8, no. 9 (September 15, 2010): 2493–2516. doi:10.3390/md8092493.

Chen, Lian, and Hengmin Cui. "Targeting Glutamine Induces Apoptosis: A Cancer Therapy Approach." *International Journal of Molecular Sciences* 16, no. 9 (September 22, 2015): 22830–55. doi:10.3390/ijms160922830.

"Collagen and Natural Gut Strings." *Massachusetts Institute of Technology.* Accessed June 14, 2016. http://web.mit.edu/3.082/www/team1_f02/collagen.htm

Dalvi, Siddhartha, Ngoc On, Hieu Nguyen, Michael Pogorzelec, Donald W. Miller, and Grant M. Hatch. "The Blood Brain Barrier—Regulation of Fatty Acid and Drug Transport." In *Neurochemistry*, Ed. Thomas Heibockel. InTech, 2014. doi:10.5772/57604. Available from: http://www.intechopen.com/books/neurochemistry/the-blood-brain-barrier-regulation-of-fatty-acid-and-drug-transport

Damiano, Rocco, Giuseppe Quarto, Ilaria Bava, Giuseppe Ucciero, Renato De Domenico, Michele I. Palumbo, and Riccardo Autorino. "Prevention of Recurrent Urinary Tract Infections by Intravesical Administration of Hyaluronic Acid and Chondroitin Sulphate: A Placebo-Controlled Randomised Trial." *European Urology* 59, no. 4 (April 2011): 645–51. doi:10.1016/j.eururo.2010.12.039.

De Vadder, Filipe, Petia Kovatcheva-Datchary, Daisy Goncalves, Jennifer Vinera, Carine Zitoun, Adeline Duchampt, Fredrik Bäckhed, et al. "Microbiota-Generated Metabolites Promote Metabolic Benefits via Gut-Brain Neural Circuits." *Cell* 156, no. 1-2 (January 2014): 84–96. doi:10.1016/j.cell.2013.12.016.

De Vita, Davide, and Salvatore Giordano. "Effectiveness of Intravesical Hyaluronic Acid/Chondroitin Sulfate in Recurrent Bacterial Cystitis: A Randomized Study." *International Urogynecology Journal* 23, no. 12 (May 22, 2012): 1707–13. doi:10.1007/s00192-012-1794-z.

Deters, Alexandra, Frank Petereit, Jörg Schmidgall, and Andreas Hensel. "N-Acetyl-D-Glucosamine Oligosaccharides Induce Mucin Secretion from Colonic Tissue and Induce Differentiation of Human Keratinocytes." *Journal of Pharmacy and Pharmacology* 60, no. 2 (February 2008): 197–204. doi:10.1211/jpp.60.2.0008.

Durie, B. G., B. Soehnlen, and J. F. Prudden. "Antitumor Activity of Bovine Cartilage Extract (Catrix-S) in the Human Tumor Stem Cell Assay." *Journal of Biological Response Modifiers* 4, no. 6 (December 1, 1985): 590–95. http://www.ncbi.nlm.nih.gov/pubmed/4087032

Fasano, A. "Zonulin and Its Regulation of Intestinal Barrier Function: The Biological Door to Inflammation, Autoimmunity, and Cancer." *Physiological Reviews* 91, no. 1 (January 1, 2011): 151–75. doi:10.1152/physrev.00003.2008.

Forstner, J. F. "Intestinal Mucins in Health and Disease." *Digestion* 17, no. 3 (January 27, 2009): 234–63. doi:10.1159/000198115.

Garlic, P. J. "Assessment of the Safety of Glutamine and Other Amino Acids." *The Journal of Nutrition* 131, no. 9 (September 1, 2001): 2556S–2561S.

Garvan Institute of Medical Research. "Bone Fractures Can Double or Triple Mortality for up to 10 Years—Garvan Institute of Medical Research." *Health News*. July 29, 2015. http://www.garvan.org.au/news/news/bone-fractures-can-double-or-triple-mortality-for-up-to-10-years

"Glutathione." *WebMD*. 2005. http://www.webmd.com/vitamins-supplements/ingredientmono-717-GLUTATHIONE.aspx?activeIngredientId=717&activeIngredientName=GLUTATHIONE

Goebel, A., S. Buhner, R. Schedel, H. Lochs, and G. Sprotte. "Altered Intestinal Permeability in Patients with Primary Fibromyalgia and in Patients with Complex Regional Pain Syndrome." *Rheumatology* 47, no. 8 (April 29, 2008): 1223–27. doi:10.1093/rheumatology/ken140.

González-Ortiz, M., R. Medina-Santillán, E. Martínez-Abundis, and C. Reynoso von Drateln. "Effect of Glycine on Insulin Secretion and Action in Healthy First-Degree Relatives of Type 2 Diabetes Mellitus Patients." *Hormone and Metabolic Research* 33, no. 6 (June 2001): 358–60. doi:10.1055/s-2001-15421.

Herrero-Beaumont, Gabriel, José Andrés Román Ivorra, María del Carmen Trabado, Francisco Javier Blanco, Pere Benito, Emilio Martín-Mola, Javier Paulino, et al. "Glucosamine Sulfate in the Treatment of Knee Osteoarthritis Symptoms: A Randomized, Double-Blind, Placebo-Controlled Study Using Acetaminophen as a Side Comparator." *Arthritis & Rheumatism* 56, no. 2 (2007): 555–67. doi:10.1002/art.22371.

Imlay, James A. "Pathways of Oxidative Damage." *Annual Review of Microbiology* 57, no. 1 (October 2003): 395–418. doi:10.1146/annurev.micro.57.030502.090938.

Insel, Thomas. "Antidepressants: A Complicated Picture." *Director's Blog*. October 29, 2015. http://www.nimh.nih.gov/about/director/2011/antidepressants-a-complicated-picture.shtml

Jaksic, Tom, David A. Wagner, John F. Burke, and Vernon R. Young. "Plasma Proline Kinetics and the Regulation of Proline Synthesis in Man." *Metabolism* 36, no. 11 (November 1987): 1040–46. doi:10.1016/0026-0495(87)90023-0.

Kasai, Kikuo, Masami Kobayashi, and Shin-Ichi Shimoda. "Stimulatory Effect of Glycine on Human Growth Hormone Secretion." *Metabolism* 27, no. 2 (February 1978): 201–8. doi:10.1016/0026-0495(78)90165-8.

Kawada, Chinatsu, Takushi Yoshida, Hideto Yoshida, Ryosuke Matsuoka, Wakako Sakamoto, Wataru Odanaka, Toshihide Sato, et al. "Ingested Hyaluronan Moisturizes Dry Skin." *Nutrition Journal* 13, no. 70 (2014). doi:10.1186/1475-2891-13-70.

Kiefer, David. "Glutathione: Uses and Risks." *WebMD*. June 15, 2015. http://www.webmd.com/vitamins-and-supplements/glutathione-uses-risks

Knuutinen, A., N. Kokkonen, J. Risteli, K. Vähäkangas, M. Kallioinen, T. Salo, T. Sorsa, et al. "Smoking Affects Collagen Synthesis and Extracellular Matrix Turnover in Human Skin." *The British Journal of Dermatology* 146, no. 4 (April 23, 2002): 588–94. doi: 10.1046/j.1365-2133.2002.04694.x

Krane, Stephen M. "The Importance of Proline Residues in the Structure, Stability and Susceptibility to Proteolytic Degradation of Collagens." *Amino Acids* 35, no. 4 (April 23, 2008): 703–10. doi:10.1007/s00726-008-0073-2.

Krishna Rao, Radha. "Role of Glutamine in Protection of Intestinal Epithelial Tight Junctions." *Journal of Epithelial Biology and Pharmacology* 5, no. 1 (January 16, 2012): 47–54. doi:10.2174/1875044301205010047.

Krishnan, Navasona, Martin B. Dickman, and Donald F. Becker. "Proline Modulates the Intracellular Redox Environment and Protects Mammalian Cells Against Oxidative Stress." *Free Radical Biology and Medicine* 44, no. 4 (February 2008): 671–81. doi:10.1016/j.freeradbiomed.2007.10.054.

Kucuktulu, Eda, Ali Guner, Izzettin Kahraman, Murat Topbas, and Uzer Kucuktulu. "The Protective Effects of Glutamine on Radiation-Induced Diarrhea." *Supportive Care in Cancer* 21, no. 4 (October 14, 2012): 1071–75. doi:10.1007/s00520-012-1627-0.

Lacey, Janet M., and Douglas W. Wilmore. "Is Glutamine a Conditionally Essential Amino Acid?" *Nutrition Reviews* 48, no. 8 (April 27, 2009): 297–309. doi:10.1111/j.1753-4887.1990.tb02967.x.

Laviano, A., A. Molfino, M. T. Lacaria, A. Canelli, S. De Leo, I. Preziosa, and F. Rossi Fanelli. "Glutamine Supplementation Favors Weight Loss in Nondieting Obese Female Patients. A Pilot Study." *European Journal of Clinical Nutrition* 68, no. 11 (September 17, 2014): 1264–66. doi:10.1038/ejcn.2014.184.

López-Corcuera, B., A. Geerlings, and C. Aragón. "Glycine Neurotransmitter Transporters: An Update." *Molecular Membrane Biology.* 18, no. 1 (June 9, 2001): 13–20. doi:10.1080/09687680010028762.

Loprinzi, Charles L., Ralph Levitt, Debra L. Barton, Jeff A. Sloan, Pam J. Atherton, Denise J. Smith, Shaker R. Dakhil, et al. "Evaluation of Shark Cartilage in Patients with Advanced Cancer." *Cancer* 104, no. 1 (2005): 176–82. doi:10.1002/cncr.21107.

Louin, G., N. Neveux, L. Cynober, M. Plotkine, C. Marchand-Leroux, and M. Jafarian-Tehrani. "Plasma Concentrations of Arginine and Related Amino Acids Following Traumatic Brain Injury: Proline as a Promising Biomarker of Brain Damage Severity." *Nitric Oxide* 17, no. 2 (September 2007): 91–97. doi:10.1016/j.niox.2007.05.006.

Maintz, Laura, and Natalija Novak. "Histamine and Histamine Intolerance." *The American Journal of Clinical Nutrition* 85, no. 5 (May 2007): 1185–96. http://ajcn.nutrition.org/content/85/5/1185.full

Mauras, N., D. Xing, L. A. Fox, K. Englert, and D. Darmaun. "Effects of Glutamine on Glycemic Control During and After Exercise in Adolescents with Type 1 Diabetes: A Pilot Study." *Diabetes Care* 33, no. 9 (June 28, 2010): 1951–53. doi:10.2337/dc10-0275.

Mayer, Emeran A. "Gut Feelings: The Emerging Biology of Gut–brain Communication." *Nature Reviews Neuroscience* 12, no. 8 (July 13, 2011): 453–66. doi:10.1038/nrn3071.

McAlindon, Timothy E., Michael P. LaValley, Juan P. Gulin, and David T. Felson. "Glucosamine and Chondroitin for Treatment of Osteoarthritis." *The Journal of the American Medical Association* 283, no. 11 (March 15, 2000): 1469–75. doi:10.1001/jama.283.11.1469.

McCance, R. A., W. Sheldon, and E. M. Widdowson. "Bone and Vegetable Broth." *Archives of Disease in Childhood* 9, no. 52 (August 1, 1934): 251–58. doi:10.1136/adc.9.52.251.

McIntosh, James, and Helen Webberley. "What Is Collagen? What Does Collagen Do?" *Medical News Today*. August 5, 2015. http://www.medicalnewstoday.com/articles/262881.php

Meléndez-Hevia, Enrique, Patricia de Paz-Lugo, Athel Cornish-Bowden, and María Luz Cárdenas. "A Weak Link in Metabolism: The Metabolic Capacity for Glycine Biosynthesis Does Not Satisfy the Need for Collagen Synthesis." *Journal of Biosciences* 34, no. 6 (December 2009): 853–72. doi:10.1007/s12038-009-0100-9.

Miyamoto, K., N. Tanaka, K. Moriguchi, R. Ueno, K. Kadomatsu, H. Kitagawa, and S. Kusunoki. "Chondroitin 6-O-Sulfate Ameliorates Experimental Autoimmune Encephalomyelitis." *Glycobiology* 24, no. 5 (February 28, 2014): 469–75. doi:10.1093/glycob/cwu014.

Morell, Sally Fallon, and Kaayla T. Daniel. *Nourishing Broth: An Old-Fashioned Remedy for the Modern World*. New York: Grand Central Life & Style, 2014.

Moskowitz, Richard J. "Cellulite." *MedlinePlus Medical Encyclopedia*. February 12, 2014. https://www.nlm.nih.gov/medlineplus/ency/article/002033.htm

Murphy, J. M., S. J. Murch, and R. O. Ball. "Proline Is Synthesized from Glutamate During Intragastric Infusion but Not During Intravenous Infusion in Neonatal Piglets." *Journal of Nutrition* 126, no. 4 (April 1996): 878–86.

National Center for Biotechnology Information. "DL-Proline." *PubChem*. September 16, 2004. Accessed May 20, 2016. http://pubchem.ncbi.nlm.nih.gov/compound/614#section=Top

National Center for Complementary and Integrative Health. "Questions and Answers: NIH Glucosamine/Chondroitin Arthritis Intervention Trial Primary Study." March 16, 2016. Accessed June 14, 2016. https://nccih.nih.gov/research/results/gait/qa.htm#moreinfo

National Institutes of Health. "Dietary Supplements." *U.S. Department of Health & Human Services*. June 24, 2011. https://ods.od.nih.gov/factsheets/DietarySupplements-HealthProfessional/#h3

National Institutes of Health: Center for Technology. *Towards Psychobiotics: The Microbiome as a Key Regulator of Brain and Behavior* [video]. *NIH VideoCasting and Podcasting.* October 6, 2015. https://videocast.nih.gov/summary.asp?Live=17162&bhcp=1

National Osteoporosis Foundation. "What Is Osteoporosis and What Causes It?" Accessed June 2016. https://www.nof.org/patients/what-is-osteoporosis/

Navarro, Sandi L., Emily White, Elizabeth D. Kantor, Yuzheng Zhang, Junghyun Rho, Xiaoling Song, Ginger L. Milne, et al. "Randomized Trial of Glucosamine and Chondroitin Supplementation on Inflammation and Oxidative Stress Biomarkers and Plasma Proteomics Profiles in Healthy Humans." *PLOS ONE* 10, no. 2 (February 26, 2015): e0117534. doi:10.1371/journal.pone.0117534.

Nelms, Marcia, Kathryn P. Sucher, Karen Lacey, and Sara Long Roth. *Nutrition Therapy and Pathophysiology.* 2nd ed. Belmont, CA: Brooks/Cole Cengage Learning, 2011.

Nelson, F. R., R. A. Zvirbulis, B. Zonca, K. W. Li, S. M. Turner, M. Pasierb, P. Wilton, et al. "Erratum to: The Effects of an Oral Preparation Containing Hyaluronic Acid (Oralvisc®) on Obese Knee Osteoarthritis Patients Determined by Pain, Function, Bradykinin, Leptin, Inflammatory Cytokines, and Heavy Water Analyses." *Rheumatology International* 35, no. 1 (July 2, 2014): 53. doi:10.1007/s00296-014-3078-z.

Nimni, Marcel E., Bo Han, and Fabiola Cordoba. "Are We Getting Enough Sulfur in Our Diet?" *Nutrition & Metabolism* 4, no. 1 (2007): 24. doi:10.1186/1743-7075-4-24.

Nunes Santiago, Amanda, Vilma Aparecida Ferreira de Godoi-Gazola, Mariana Fachin Milani, Vanessa Cristina de Campos, Vanessa Rodrigues Vilela, Maria Montserrat Diaz Pedrosa, and Roberto Barbosa Bazotte. "Oral Glutamine Is Superior Than Oral Glucose to Promote Glycemia Recovery in Mice Submitted to Insulin-Induced Hypoglycemia." *International Journal of Endocrinology* 2013 (2013): 1–7. doi:10.1155/2013/841514.

Pérez-Torres, I., A. M. Zúñiga-Muñoz, and V. G. Lans. "Beneficial Effects of the Amino Acid Glycine." *Mini Reviews in Medicinal Chemistry.* June 14, 2016. http://www.ncbi.nlm.nih.gov/pubmed/27292783.

Praveen, Mamidipudi R., Archana Koul, Abhay R. Vasavada, Deepak Pandita, Nirmit V. Dixit, and Farida F. Dahodwala. "DisCoVisc Versus the Soft-Shell Technique Using Viscoat and Provisc in Phacoemulsification: Randomized Clinical Trial." *Journal of Cataract & Refractive Surgery* 34, no. 7 (July 2008): 1145–51. doi:10.1016/j.jcrs.2008.03.019.

Prudden, John F. "The Treatment of Human Cancer with Agents Prepared from Bovine Cartilage." *Journal of Biological Response Modifiers* 4, no. 6 (December 1985): 551–84.

Prudden, John F., and Leslie L. Balassa. "The Biological Activity of Bovine Cartilage Preparations." *Seminars in Arthritis and Rheumatism* 3, no. 4 (June 1974): 287–321. doi:10.1016/0049-0172(74)90003-1.

Reeds, P. "Dispensable and Indispensable Amino Acids for Humans." *Journal of Nutrition* 130, no. 7 (July 2000): 1835–40. http://jn.nutrition.org/content/130/7/1835S.full

Rennard, Barbara O., Ronald F. Ertl, Gail L. Gossman, Richard A. Robbins, and Stephen I. Rennard. "Chicken Soup Inhibits Neutrophil Chemotaxis in Vitro." *Chest* 118, no. 4 (October 2000): 1150–57. doi:10.1378/chest.118.4.1150.

Richter, J., K. Capková, V. Hříbalová, L. Vannucci, I. Danyi, M. Malý, and A. Fišerová. "Collagen-Induced Arthritis: Severity and Immune Response Attenuation Using Multivalent N-Acetyl Glucosamine." *Clinical and Experimental Immunology* 177, no. 1 (March 5, 2014): 121–33. doi: 10.1111/cei.12313.

Riordan, S. M., C. J. McIver, D. H. Thomas, V. M. Duncombe, T. D. Bolin, and M. C. Thomas. "Luminal Bacteria and Small-Intestinal Permeability." *Scandinavian Journal of Gastroenterology* 32, no. 6 (January 1997): 556–63. doi:10.3109/00365529709025099.

Rohrmann, Sabine, and Jakob Linseisen. "Processed Meat: The Real Villain?" *Proceedings of the Nutrition Society* 75, no. 3 (December 1, 2015): 233–41. doi:10.1017/s0029665115004255.

Rosen, H. N., H. Salemme, A. J. Zeind, A. C. Moses, A. Shapiro, and S. L. Greenspan. "Chicken Soup Revisited: Calcium Content of Soup Increases with Duration of Cooking." *Calcified Tissue International* 54, no. 6 (June 1994): 486–88. doi:10.1007/bf00334329.

Saito, M., and K. Marumo. "Collagen Cross-Links as a Determinant of Bone Quality: A Possible Explanation for Bone Fragility in Aging, Osteoporosis, and Diabetes Mellitus." *Osteoporosis International* 21, no. 2 (September 17, 2009): 195–214. doi:10.1007/s00198-009-1066-z.

Salvatore, S., R. Heuschkel, S. Tomlin, S. E. Davies, S. Edwards, J. A. Walker-Smith, I. French, et al. "A Pilot Study of N-Acetyl Glucosamine, a Nutritional Substrate for Glycosaminoglycan Synthesis, in Paediatric Chronic Inflammatory Bowel Disease." *Alimentary Pharmacology & Therapeutics* 14, no. 12 (December 21, 2000): 1567–79. doi: 10.1046/j.1365-2036.2000.00883.x.

Sanz, A. "Methionine Restriction Decreases Mitochondrial Oxygen Radical Generation and Leak as Well as Oxidative Damage to Mitochondrial DNA and Proteins." *The FASEB Journal* 20, no. 8 (June 1, 2006): 1064–73. doi:10.1096/fj.05-5568com.

Schneider, Heinz, Emmanuel Maheu, and Michel Cucherat. "Symptom-Modifying Effect of Chondroitin Sulfate in Knee Osteoarthritis: A Meta-Analysis of Randomized Placebo-Controlled Trials Performed with Structum®." *The Open Rheumatology Journal* 6, no. 1 (July 25, 2012): 183–89. doi:10.2174/1874312901206010183.

Schneider, Michael J., David M. Brady, and Stephen M. Perle. "Commentary: Differential Diagnosis of Fibromyalgia Syndrome: Proposal of a Model and Algorithm for Patients Presenting with the Primary Symptom of Chronic Widespread Pain." *Journal of Manipulative and Physiological Therapeutics* 29, no. 6 (July 2006): 493–501. doi:10.1016/j.jmpt.2006.06.010.

Schuette, K. "Stock vs Broth: Are You Confused?" *Gaps Info*, March 2012. Accessed May 12, 2016. http://www.gapsinfo.com/wp-content/uploads/2012/03/Stock-vs.-Broth.pdf

SELFNutritionData. "Foods Highest in Glycine." 2014. Accessed May 7, 2016. http://nutritiondata.self.com/foods-000094000000000000000.html

SELFNutritionData. "Foods Highest in Proline." 2014. Accessed May 7, 2016. http://nutritiondata.self.com/foods-000095000000000000000.html

Seyfried, T. N., R. E. Flores, A. M. Poff, and D. P. D'Agostino. "Cancer as a Metabolic Disease: Implications for Novel Therapeutics." *Carcinogenesis* 35, no. 3 (December 16, 2013): 515–27. doi:10.1093/carcin/bgt480.

Shaughnessy, Allen F. "Chondroitin/Glucosamine Equal to Celecoxib for Knee Osteoarthritis." *American Family Physician* 93, no. 12 (June 15, 2016). http://www.aafp.org/afp/2016/0615/p1032.html

Sonnenburg, Justin, and Erica Sonnenburg. *The Good Gut: Taking Control of Your Weight, Your Mood, and Your Long-Term Health.* New York: Penguin Books, 2015.

Spencer, Thomas E., Guoyao Wu, Fuller W. Bazer, Robert C. Burghardt, Gregory A. Johnson, Carey M. Satterfield, Darrell A. Knabe, et al. "Reference Tools." *Amino Acids* 40, no. 4 (August 10, 2010): 1053–63. doi:10.1007/s00726-010-0715-z.

Sugiyama, Kimio, Yasuo Kushima, and Keiichiro Muramatsu. "Effect of Dietary Glycine on Methionine Metabolism in Rats Fed a High-Methionine Diet." *Journal of Nutritional Science and Vitaminology* 33, no. 3 (1987): 195–205. doi:10.3177/jnsv.33.195.

Takahashi, H., M. Ohara, and K. Imai. "Collagen Diseases with Gastrointestinal Manifestations." *Japanese Journal of Clinical Immunology* 27, no. 3 (August 5, 2004): 145–55. http://www.ncbi.nlm.nih.gov/pubmed/15291251

Tertov, V. V., A. N. Orekhov, I. A. Sobenin, J. D. Morrisett, A. M. Gotto, and J. G. Guevara. "Carbohydrate Composition of Protein and Lipid Components in Sialic Acid-Rich and-Poor Low Density Lipoproteins from Subjects with and Without Coronary Artery Disease." *Journal of Lipid Research* 34, no. 3 (March 1993): 365–75. http://www.jlr.org/content/34/3/365.full.pdf+html

Therapeutic Research Center. "Chondroitin Sulfate." *Natural Medicines.* Accessed June 14, 2016. https://naturalmedicines.therapeuticresearch.com/databases/food,-herbs-supplements/professional.aspx?productid=744

Therapeutic Research Center. "Hyaluronic Acid." *Natural Medicines.* 2016. Accessed June 14, 2016. https://naturalmedicines.therapeuticresearch.com/databases/food,-herbs-supplements/professional.aspx?productid=1062

Therapeutic Research Center. "Natural Medicines Database." *Natural Medicines.* 2016. Accessed May 30, 2016. https://naturalmedicines.therapeuticresearch.com/databases/food,-herbs-supplements/professional.aspx?productid=878

Trentham, D. E., R. A. Dynesius-Trentham, E. J. Orav, D. Combitchi, C. Lorenzo, K. L. Sewell, D. A. Hafler, et al. "Effects of Oral Administration of Type II Collagen on Rheumatoid Arthritis." *Science* 261, no. 5129 (September 24, 1993): 1727–30. doi: 10.1126/science.8378772.

U.S. DA. "DRI Nutrient Reports." *National Agricultural Library.* August 2016. http://fnic.nal.usda.gov/dietary-guidance/dietary-reference-intakes/dri-nutrient-reports

U.S. FDA. "Information for Healthcare Professionals: Celecoxib (marketed as Celebrex)." August 13, 2013. Accessed June 2016. http://www.fda.gov/Drugs/DrugSafety/PostmarketDrugSafetyInformationforPatientsandProviders/ucm124655.htm

Vigier, Sylvain, Christophe Helary, Olivia Fromigue, Pierre Marie, and Marie-Madeleine Giraud-Guille. "Collagen Supramolecular and Suprafibrillar Organizations on Osteoblasts Long-Term Behavior: Benefits for Bone Healing Materials." *Journal of Biomedical Materials Research* 94A, no. 2 (2010): 556–67. doi:10.1002/jbm.a.32717.

Wang, Weiwei, Zhenlong Wu, Zhaolai Dai, Ying Yang, Junjun Wang, and Guoyao Wu. "Glycine Metabolism in Animals and Humans: Implications for Nutrition and Health." *Amino Acids* 45, no. 3 (April 25, 2013): 463–77. doi:10.1007/s00726-013-1493-1.

Wang, X., X. Shen, X. Li, and C. Mauli Agrawal. "Age-Related Changes in the Collagen Network and Toughness of Bone." *Bone* 31, no. 1 (July 2002): 1–7. doi:10.1016/s8756-3282(01)00697-4.

Womack, Madelyn, and William Rose. "The Role of Proline, Hydroxyproline, and Glutamic Acid in Growth." *Journal of Biological Chemistry* 171, no. 1 (July 24, 1947): 37–50. http://www.jbc.org/content/171/1/37.short

Xie, Qingwen, Rong Shi, Gang Xu, Lifu Cheng, Liyun Shao, and Jianyu Rao. "Effects of AR7 Joint Complex on Arthralgia for Patients with Osteoarthritis: Results of a Three-Month Study in Shanghai, China." *Nutrition Journal* 7, no. 31 (2008): 1–6. doi:10.1186/1475-2891-7-31.

Yamadera, Wataru, Kentaro Inagawa, Shintaro Chiba, Makoto Bannai, Michio Takahaski, and Kazuhiko Nakayama. "Glycine Ingestion Improves Subjective Sleep Quality in Human Volunteers, Correlating with Polysomnographic Changes." *Sleep and Biological Rhythms* 5, no. 2 (March 27, 2007): 126–31. doi:10.1111/j.1479-8425.2007.00262.x.

Young, A. M. J., and H. F. Bradford. "Excitatory Amino Acid Neurotransmitters in the Corticostriate Pathway: Studies Using Intracerebral Microdialysis in Vivo." *Journal of Neurochemistry* 47, no. 5 (November 1986): 1399–1404. doi:10.1111/j.1471-4159.1986.tb00771.x.

Zhang, Ling-Ling, Wei Wei, Feng Xiao, Jian-Hua Xu, Chun-De Bao, Li-Qing Ni, and Xing-Fu Li. "A Randomized, Double-blind, Multicenter, Controlled Clinical Trial of Chicken Type II Collagen in Patients with Rheumatoid Arthritis." *Arthritis & Rheumatism* 59, no. 7 (July 15, 2008): 905–10. doi:10.1002/art.23824.

Zhang, Yanlu, Zheng Gang Zhang, Michael Chopp, Yuling Meng, Li Zhang, Asim Mahmood, and Ye Xiong. "Treatment of Traumatic Brain Injury in Rats with N-Acetyl-Seryl-Aspartyl-Lysyl-Proline." *Journal of Neurosurgery* (May 20, 2016): 1–14. doi:10.3171/2016.3.jns152699.

Zhu, Andy, Ishita Patel, Melinda Hidalgo, and Veeral Ghandi. "N-Acetylglucosamine for Treatment of Inflammatory Bowel Disease." *Natural Medicine Journal* 7, no. 4 (April 2015). http://www.naturalmedicinejournal.com/journal/2015-04/n-acetylglucosamine-treatment-inflammatory-bowel-disease

Chapter 4. Digging Deeper

Daniel, Kaayla. "Bone Broth and Lead Contamination: A Very Flawed Study in Medical Hypotheses." *Weston A. Price Foundation*. March 12, 2013. Accessed May 15, 2016. http://www.westonaprice.org/health-topics/soy-alert/bone-broth-and-lead-contamination-a-very-flawed-study-in-medical-hypotheses/

Krishnan, Navasona, Martin B. Dickman, and Donald F. Becker. "Proline Modulates the Intracellular Redox Environment and Protects Mammalian Cells Against Oxidative

Stress." *Free Radical Biology and Medicine* 44, no. 4 (February 2008): 671–81. doi:10.1016/j. freeradbiomed.2007.10.054.

Monro, J. A., R. Leon, and B. K. Puri. "The Risk of Lead Contamination in Bone Broth Diets." *Medical Hypotheses* 80, no. 4 (April 2013): 389–90. doi:10.1016/j.mehy.2012.12.026.

National Institutes of Health. "Dietary Supplements." *Office of Dietary Supplements: Health Information*. June 24, 2011. https://ods.od.nih.gov/factsheets/DietarySupplements-HealthProfessional/#h3

Seneff, Stephanie, and Anthony Samsel. "Glyphosate, Pathways to Modern Diseases III: Manganese, Neurological Diseases, and Associated Pathologies." *Surgical Neurology International* 6, no. 45 (2015). doi:10.4103/2152-7806.153876.

U.S. EPA. "Basic Information about Lead in Drinking Water." March 17, 2016. Accessed May 10, 2016. https://www.epa.gov/ground-water-and-drinking-water/basic-information-about-lead-drinking-water#regs

"What Is Glyphosate?" Monsanto. 2014. http://www.monsanto.com/sitecollectiondocuments/glyphosate-safety-health.pdf

Chapter 5. Ancestral Diet Overview

Carrera-Bastos, Pedro, Maelan Fontes-Villalba, James H. O'Keefe, Staffan Lindeberg, and Loren Cordain. "The Western Diet and Lifestyle and Diseases of Civilization." *Research Reports in Clinical Cardiology* 2011, no. 2 (March 9, 2011): 15–35. doi:10.2147/rrcc.s16919.

Cordain, L., S. B. Eaton, J. Brand Miller, N. Mann, and K. Hill. "The Paradoxical Nature of Hunter-Gatherer Diets: Meat-Based, yet Non-Atherogenic." *European Journal of Clinical Nutrition* 56, no. s1 (March 18, 2002): S42–S52. doi:10.1038/sj.ejcn.1601353.

Frassetto, L. A., M. Schloetter, M. Mietus-Synder, R. C. Morris, and A. Sebastian. "Metabolic and Physiologic Improvements from Consuming a Paleolithic, Hunter-Gatherer Type Diet." *European Journal of Clinical Nutrition* 63, no. 8 (February 11, 2009): 947–55. doi:10.1038/ejcn.2009.4.

Hyman, Mark. *Eat Fat, Get Thin: Why the Fat We Eat Is the Key to Sustained Weight Loss and Vibrant Health*. New York: Little, Brown and Company, 2016.

Jönsson, Tommy, Yvonne Granfeldt, Bo Ahrén, Ulla-Carin Branell, Gunvor Pålsson, Anita Hansson, Margareta Söderström, et al. "Beneficial Effects of a Paleolithic Diet on Cardiovascular Risk Factors in Type 2 Diabetes: A Randomized Cross-over Pilot Study." *Cardiovascular Diabetology* 8, no. 1 (2009): 35. doi:10.1186/1475-2840-8-35.

Konner, M., and S. B. Eaton. "Paleolithic Nutrition: Twenty-Five Years Later." *Nutrition in Clinical Practice* 25, no. 6 (December 1, 2010): 594–602. doi:10.1177/0884533610385702.

Kowalski, L. M. and J. Bujko. "Evaluation of Biological and Clinical Potential of Paleolithic Diet." *Roczniki Państwowego Zakładu Higieny* 63, no. 1 (2012): 9–15. http://wydawnictwa.pzh.gov.pl/roczniki_pzh/ocena-potencjalu-biologicznego-i-klinicznego-diety-paleolitycznej?lang=en

Lindeberg, S., T. Jönsson, Y. Granfeldt, E. Borgstrand, J. Soffman, K. Sjöström, and B. Ahrén. "A Palaeolithic Diet Improves Glucose Tolerance More Than a Mediterranean-Like Diet in Individuals with Ischaemic Heart Disease." *Diabetologia* 50, no. 9 (June 22, 2007): 1795–1807. doi:10.1007/s00125-007-0716-y.

Manheimer, E. W., E. J. van Zuuren, Z. Fedorowicz, and H. Pijl. "Paleolithic Nutrition for Metabolic Syndrome: Systematic Review and Meta-Analysis." *American Journal of Clinical Nutrition* 102, no. 4 (August 12, 2015): 922–32. doi:10.3945/ajcn.115.113613.

Nordmann, A. J., A. Nordmann, M. Briel, U. Keller, W. S. Yancy, B. J. Brehm, and H. C. Bucher. "Effects of Low-Carbohydrate Vs Low-Fat Diets on Weight Loss and Cardiovascular Risk Factors: A Meta-Analysis of Randomized Controlled Trials." *Archives of Internal Medicine* 166, no. 3 (February 13, 2006): 285–93. doi:10.1001/archinte.166.3.285.

Österdahl, M., T. Kocturk, A. Koochek, and P. E. Wändell. "Effects of a Short-Term Intervention with a Paleolithic Diet in Healthy Volunteers." *European Journal of Clinical Nutrition* 62, no. 5 (May 16, 2007): 682–85. doi:10.1038/sj.ejcn.1602790.

"Part D. Ch 1: Food and Nutrient Intakes, and Health: Current Status and Trends." In *Scientific Report of the 2015 Dietary Guidelines Advisory Committee. Health.gov*. September 6, 2015. Accessed June 5, 2016. http://health.gov/dietaryguidelines/2015-scientific-report/06-chapter-1/d1-2.asp

Ryberg, M., S. Sandberg, C. Mellberg, O. Stegle, B. Lindahl, C. Larsson, J. Hauksson, et al. "A Palaeolithic-Type Diet Causes Strong Tissue-Specific Effects on Ectopic Fat Deposition in Obese Postmenopausal Women." *Journal of Internal Medicine* 274, no. 1 (March 11, 2013): 67–76. doi:10.1111/joim.12048.

Sonnenburg, Justin, and Erica Sonnenburg. *The Good Gut: Taking Control of Your Weight, Your Mood, and Your Long-Term Health*. New York: Penguin Books, 2015.

Spreadbury, Ian. "Comparison with Ancestral Diets Suggests Dense Acellular Carbohydrates Promote an Inflammatory Microbiota, and May Be the Primary Dietary Cause of Leptin Resistance and Obesity." *Diabetes, Metabolic Syndrome and Obesity: Targets and Therapy* 2012, no. 5 (July 6, 2012): 175–89. doi:10.2147/dmso.s33473.

Teicholz, Nina. *The Big Fat Surprise: Why Butter, Meat, and Cheese Belong in a Healthy Diet*. New York: Simon & Schuster Paperbacks, 2014.

Chapter 6. Ancestral Lifestyle

Andrews, R. C., O. Herlihy, D. E. Livingstone, R. Andrew, and B. R. Walker. "Abnormal Cortisol Metabolism and Tissue Sensitivity to Cortisol in Patients with Glucose Intolerance." *The Journal of Clinical Endocrinology and Metabolism* 87, no. 12 (December 6, 2002): 5587–93. doi: 10.1210/jc.2002-020048.

Bauman, Adrian, Barbara E. Ainsworth, James F. Sallis, Maria Hagströmer, Cora L. Craig, Fiona C. Bull, Michael Pratt, et al. "The Descriptive Epidemiology of Sitting." *American Journal of Preventive Medicine* 41, no. 2 (August 2011): 228–35. doi:10.1016/j.amepre.2011.05.003.

"Body Burden: The Pollution in Newborns." *Environmental Working Group*. July 14, 2005. Accessed June 2016. http://www.ewg.org/research/body-burden-pollution-newborns.

"Britons Spend More Than 14 Hours a Day Sitting Down." *The Telegraph*. May 19, 2010. http://www.telegraph.co.uk/news/health/news/7738663/Britons-spend-more-than-14-hours-a-day-sitting-down.html

Brooks, K. A., and J. G. Carter. "Overtraining, Exercise, and Adrenal Insufficiency." *Journal of Novel Physiotherapies* 3, no. 1 (2013). doi:10.4172/2165-7025.1000125.

Carrera-Bastos, Pedro, Maelan Fontes-Villalba, James H. O'Keefe, Staffan Lindeberg, and Loren Cordain. "The Western Diet and Lifestyle and Diseases of Civilization." *Research Reports in Clinical Cardiology* 2011, no. 2 (March 9, 2011): 15–35. doi:10.2147/rrcc.s16919.

Chang, Anne-Marie, Daniel Aeschbach, Jeanne F. Duffy, and Charles A. Czeisler. "Evening Use of Light-Emitting EReaders Negatively Affects Sleep, Circadian Timing, and Next-Morning Alertness." *Proceedings of the National Academy of Sciences* 112, no. 4 (December 22, 2014): 1232–37. doi:10.1073/pnas.1418490112.

Elenkov, Ilia J., Elizabeth L. Webster, David J. Torpy, and George P. Chrousos. "Stress, Corticotropin-Releasing Hormone, Glucocorticoids, and the Immune/inflammatory Response: Acute and Chronic Effects." *Annals of the New York Academy of Sciences* 876, no. 1 (June 1999): 1–13. doi:10.1111/j.1749-6632.1999.tb07618.x.

Epel, E., R. Lapidus, B. McEwen, and K. Brownell. "Stress May Add Bite to Appetite in Women: A Laboratory Study of Stress-Induced Cortisol and Eating Behavior." *Psychoneuroendocrinology* 26, no. 1: 37–49. doi: http://dx.doi.org/10.1016/S0306-4530(00)00035-4.

Epel, E. S., B. McEwen, T. Seeman, K. Matthews, G. Castellazzo, K. D. Brownell, J. Bell, and J. R. Ickovics. "Stress and Body Shape: Stress-Induced Cortisol Secretion Is Consistently Greater Among Women with Central Fat." *Psychosomatic Medicine*. 62, no. 5 (October 6, 2000): 623–32. http://journals.lww.com/psychosomaticmedicine/Abstract/2000/09000/Stress_and_Body_Shape__Stress_Induced_Cortisol.5.aspx

Genuis, Stephen J. "Sensitivity-Related Illness: The Escalating Pandemic of Allergy, Food Intolerance and Chemical Sensitivity." *Science of the Total Environment* 408, no. 24 (November 2010): 6047–61. doi:10.1016/j.scitotenv.2010.08.047.

Hill, E. E., E. Zack, C. Battaglini, M. Viru, and A. C. Hackney. "Exercise and Circulating Cortisol Levels: The Intensity Threshold Effect." *Journal of Endocrinological Investigation*. 31, no. 7 (September 13, 2008): 587–91. http://link.springer.com/article/10.1007/BF03345606

Hodges, Romilly E., and Deanna M. Minich. "Modulation of Metabolic Detoxification Pathways Using Foods and Food-Derived Components: A Scientific Review with Clinical Application." *Journal of Nutrition and Metabolism* 2015 (2015): 1–23. doi:10.1155/2015/760689.

Katerndahl, D. A., I. R. Bell, R. F. Palmer, and C. S. Miller. "Chemical Intolerance in Primary Care Settings: Prevalence, Comorbidity, and Outcomes." *The Annals of Family Medicine* 10, no. 4 (July 1, 2012): 357–65. doi:10.1370/afm.1346.

Nelms, Marcia, Kathryn P. Sucher, Karen Lacey, and Sara Long Roth. *Nutrition Therapy and Pathophysiology*. 2nd ed. Belmont, CA: Brooks/Cole Cengage Learning, 2011.

Nordmann, A. J., A. Nordmann, M. Briel, U. Keller, W. S. Yancy, B. J. Brehm, and H. C. Bucher. "Effects of Low-Carbohydrate vs Low-Fat Diets on Weight Loss and Cardiovascular Risk

Factors: A Meta-Analysis of Randomized Controlled Trials." *Archives of Internal Medicine*. 166, no. 3 (February 16, 2006): 285–93. doi:10.1001/archinte.166.3.285.

Patel, A. V., L. Bernstein, A. Deka, H. S. Feigelson, P. T. Campbell, S. M. Gapstur, G. A. Colditz, et al. "Leisure Time Spent Sitting in Relation to Total Mortality in a Prospective Cohort of US Adults." *American Journal of Epidemiology* 172, no. 4 (July 22, 2010): 419–29. doi:10.1093/aje/kwq155.

Pizzorno, J. "Conventional Laboratory Tests to Assess Toxin Burden." *Integrative Medicine* 14, no. 5 (October 2015): 8–16. http://www.ncbi.nlm.nih.gov/pubmed/26770160

Sher, L. "Type D Personality: The Heart, Stress, and Cortisol." *QJM : Monthly Journal of the Association of Physicians*. 98, no. 5 (April 12, 2005): 323–29. doi: http://dx.doi.org/10.1093/qjmed/hci064

Weinstein, Richard. *The Stress Effect: Discover the Connection Between Stress and Disease and Reclaim Your Health*. New York: Avery, 2004.

Chapter 7. Intermittent Fasting

Bengmark, Stig. "Obesity, the Deadly Quartet and the Contribution of the Neglected Daily Organ Rest—A New Dimension of Un-Health and Its Prevention." *Hepatobiliary Surgery and Nutrition* 4, no. 4 (August 4, 2015): 278–88. doi:10.3978/j.issn.2304-3881.2015.07.02.

Patterson, Ruth E., Gail A. Laughlin, Andrea Z. LaCroix, Sheri J. Hartman, Loki Natarajan, Carolyn M. Senger, María Elena Martínez, et al. "Intermittent Fasting and Human Metabolic Health." *Journal of the Academy of Nutrition and Dietetics* 115, no. 8 (August 2015): 1203–12. doi:10.1016/j.jand.2015.02.018.

Testimonials

- I've been eating an ancestral diet since 2011, and I'm always looking for opportunities to improve my nutrition. However, as a working mom and physician, I don't have the time to read all the latest nutrition research. Erin presented a great, easy-to-follow program that was evidence-based. I felt great with the intermittent fasting and experienced a definite decrease in cravings. —Brooke, Wichita, Kansas

- I really loved the community, recipes, and encouragement of this program. I had great results from the program. My digestion totally turned around, and I was not nearly as hungry. —Jeannette

- The more structured eating schedule has also been of great benefit to improve my habits, and the easy-to-follow recipes were great. I'm not exactly a master chef, but I was very pleased with the results. I would definitely recommend to anyone looking to tighten up their way of eating and kick the easy oven meals and processed snacky items. With a little bit of extra effort and planning, these wholesome meals are worth it to feel great! —Stephen, Bury St Edmunds, United Kingdom

- This program put me on the path for real health using real food. My weight is coming off, and I am not even hungry! —Kathleen

- I was very satisfied with the program. My favorite part was the variety of recipes. The program helped me get a little more re-focused. It gave me some new, clean recipes. I'm not able to exercise right now due to an injury so this helped me feel good. I lost 5 pounds, and it helped my blood glucose levels. —Katie, O'Fallon, Missouri

- My favorite thing about the program was how easy it was to make and use. I thought all of the recipes were going to be soups. NOT! I also liked how so much was done for us: menus, shopping lists, clear instructions, and scientific background. All I had to do was make and eat it! Most importantly, I had great results. I noticed no more bloating, my skin started clearing up, and I lost weight! —Pam, Irving, Texas

- The recipes were great, and I love how liberated from food I felt on the program. I felt like I was in charge versus vulnerable to cravings and moods swings. —Rachelle, Edmond, Oklahoma

- With this program I increased my exercise and have more energy now. I have lost 2 kg (4.4 lbs) with 5 days to go. —Amanda, Normanville, South Australia

- Overall I feel so. much. better. I lost inches as well. My family likes the recipes, and I've continued to use them. When I began, I'd been nursing an injury; as I cleaned up my diet (even more), my knee felt better. I've begun a couch-to-5K running program again, and I am working out with heavier weights! —Shelly, Dallas, Texas

- The most helpful thing about this program was the bone broth and other recipes and the meal plan/shopping lists. I joined this program to support a healthy pregnancy and felt that the organized plans really helped me accomplish that. I ate the clean breakfast options instead of fasting because of pregnancy, and I felt that the addition of drinking broth at breakfast and snack was awesome. My husband actually lost a few inches! —Shanna

- My favorite things about this program were the detailed menus, shopping lists, and recipes that made the whole process a no-brainer. I do better if I know in advance each day what's for dinner and snacks. I love the recipes, and I've rediscovered the pleasures of cooking through Erin's programs. I'm starting week 3 and am down another pound, even without being 100% faithful to the program. For me, it worked best to include a clean breakfast option with my broth rather than fasting each morning. —Theta, Loomis, California

- My favorite things about this program were learning about the nutritional benefits of bone broth, learning how to make it confidently, and understanding that I can fast intermittently and exercise without feeling hungry. The only problem I had was that my family kept eating the food, so I had to be more creative on leftover meals! I am truly looking forward to what the future holds. —Emma, Bury St Edmunds, Suffolk, United Kingdom

Cooking Conversion Charts

Metric and Imperial Conversions

(These conversions are rounded for convenience)

Ingredient	Cups/ Tablespoons/ Teaspoons	Ounces	Grams/ Milliliters
Butter	1 cup/ 16 tablespoons/ 2 sticks	8 ounces	230 grams
Cheese, shredded	1 cup	4 ounces	110 grams
Fruit, dried	1 cup	4 ounces	120 grams
Fruits or veggies, chopped	1 cup	5 to 7 ounces	145 to 200 grams
Fruits or veggies, pureed	1 cup	8.5 ounces	245 grams
Honey or maple syrup	1 tablespoon	0.75 ounce	20 grams
Liquids: cream, milk, water, or juice	1 cup	8 fluid ounces	240 milliliters
Oats	1 cup	5.5 ounces	150 grams
Salt	1 teaspoon	0.2 ounce	6 grams
Spices: cinnamon, cloves, ginger, or nutmeg (ground)	1 teaspoon	0.2 ounce	5 milliliters
Vanilla extract	1 teaspoon	0.2 ounce	4 grams

Oven Temperatures

Fahrenheit	Celsius	Gas Mark
225°	110°	¼
250°	120°	½
275°	140°	1
300°	150°	2
325°	160°	3
350°	180°	4
375°	190°	5
400°	200°	6
425°	220°	7
450°	230°	8